LIVING
WITH
HEART
DISEASE

Patsy Westcott

WARD LOCK

A WARD LOCK BOOK
First published in the UK 1998
by Ward Lock
Wellington House
125 Strand
London
WC2R 0BB

A Cassell imprint

A British Library Cataloguing in Publication Data block for this book may be obtained
from the British Library

ISBN 0 7063 7666 8

Edited by Caroline Ball
Designed by Anita Ruddell
Printed and bound in Great Britain by MPG Books Ltd, Bodmin, Cornwall

CONTENTS

FOREWORD

CORONARY HEART DISEASE is not only one of the major causes of ill health, but it usually presents itself suddenly, unexpectedly and dramatically. This often leaves the sufferer and immediate family feeling stunned and anxious. What is going to happen next? Am I going to die at any moment? What does the future hold? The truth is that, following recovery, most people with coronary heart disease lead a normal and active life.

Picking up the pieces after you or someone close to you suffers a heart attack or develops angina can be difficult and demanding. This is especially true when you are dealing with something you yourself do not understand and are perhaps afraid to enquire about. The uncertainty and fear of the unknown is often worse than the reality and this only serves to increase the anxiety and to impede the healing process. This book sets out to redress this imbalance and helps you to understand and deal with the problems of living with coronary heart disease.

Patsy Westcott takes us through the basics of how the heart works and what happens during an angina or heart attack. She goes on to explain, through the experiences of real people, the variety of ways coronary heart disease affects people, how sufferers have reacted and the ways people have come to terms with their condition. Shared experiences often dispel feelings of isolation and help us to understand our own, sometimes confusing feelings.

A part of becoming ill is that you are exposed to a lot of medical jargon and undergo a battery of medical tests which may initially sound rather daunting. Patsy provides us with a clear description of each of the major investigations and the medical terms used in cardiology, the medical speciality concerned with the heart. The book goes on to lay out the various treatment options, from the humble aspirin through to major bypass surgery. Understanding the limitations, complications and the effects of each available treatment is equally important and this is explained in simple language. There is also a chapter dealing with complementary medicine, although it is important to remember that this should only be seen as 'complementary' rather than an alternative to orthodox medicine.

There are a lot of myths and misconceptions surrounding coronary heart disease. *Living with Heart Disease* attempts to dispel some of these and emphasises the important changes and treatments which can have a real impact on your subsequent health and well-being. Lifestyle changes are often the most difficult to address and recognizing the problem is the first step. Helpful hints, practical guidance and means of getting further help and assistance are all contained within the book. Having improved their diet and lifestyle, people often say that they feel much happier about themselves, not only physically but mentally as well. Indeed, some people find that life becomes even more enjoyable after their heart attack.

With the aid of modern treatments, most people with coronary heart disease lead full and rewarding lives for many years. How successful you will be is dependent on your attitude and your approach to the treatment and the necessary lifestyle changes. *Living with Heart Disease* provides you with the practical background and support to start you on your way.

Dr David Newby
Lecturer in Cardiology
The Royal Infirmary of Edinburgh

ACKNOWLEDGEMENTS

MANY PEOPLE HELPED IN THE WRITING OF THIS BOOK: doctors, nurses, psychologists, support group organizers and people with heart disease. The British Heart Foundation, and in particular Helena Hird and Belinda Linden, were tremendously helpful in answering my questions, pointing me towards sources of help and providing information and literature. Much of the information in the more 'technical' parts of the book is drawn from BHF leaflets, including the diagram on page 20. Thanks is also due to the American Heart Association for providing information and leaflets. The questionnaire 'How angry are you?' on page 119 is reprinted by permission of the authors.

Of the many experts I spoke to a special thanks is owed to Dr David Newby, lecturer in cardiology at Edinburgh University, who patiently explained to me the most recent thinking on heart disease and also read through the manuscript. Thanks is also due to Professor Bob Lewin and Professor David Thompson of the British Heart Foundation's Rehabilitation Research Unit at Hull University, to Dr Ann Williams, nutritionist at Reading University, to Dr Nicola Stuckey, psychologist at Astley Ainslie Hospital, Edinburgh, to Dr Mark McDermott, lecturer in health psychology at the University of East London and to John Lenciewicz, of the Institute of Human Sexuality.

Thanks, too, to Claire Lowe at the British Medical Association's Press Office, to the Institute of Sports Medicine Library and to Pilgrim Hospital Library in Boston. Throughout the writing of the book commissioning editor Helen Denholm of Cassell was a huge support and help. Above all, my thanks go to all those men and women who so generously shared with me their experience of heart disease. In particular I should like to mention John and Fiona of the St George's Family Support Group, Bernice and Mike of the Chester Heart Support Group, Victor of the Royal Free Hospital Support Group, Norma Jackson of the Zipper Club and Linda and Len who have helped many people set up support groups. Without them and all the people they introduced me to up and down the UK this book would not have been possible.

WHO'S WHO IN THIS BOOK

To SAVE HAVING TO REPEAT EACH PERSON'S STORY, a potted history of the main people who spoke to me is given below:

Carolyn, 41, developed angina when she was 39 and it was subsequently discovered that one artery was almost completely blocked. She has had two stents inserted. She is married with no children and works for a big plastics company.

Clive, 52, is a civil servant who took part in a famous UK study into risk factors for heart disease called the Whitehall Study. He developed silent ischaemia and high blood pressure, and subsequently suffered a heart attack. He has since returned to work.

Gill, 50, is a former manager in a big national company. She started to experience angina and other symptoms of heart disease when she was 47 and had a double bypass a year later. Three months after the bypass she developed a blood clot on her bowel. Although she returned to work briefly for two mornings a week following her initial surgery, she has since decided to take early retirement.

Greta is 52. A long-standing diabetic, dependent on insulin, she developed angina when she was 40. A year later she had a bypass operation. She runs a heart support group.

Howard, 60, is a former university lecturer. He was 56 when he developed angina. Two and a half years later he was admitted to hospital for a bypass. He returned to work but has now retired.

Jim is 67. He had a mild heart attack when he was 55 and a triple bypass operation three years later. He returned to his job in middle management in industry but subsequently left and went to work for a charity. Today he is retired.

John, 48, is a former chef. He developed intermittent claudication (leg cramps caused by furred arteries) when he was 36 and subsequently suffered a silent heart attack. He has had two bypass operations. He now works as a painter/decorator, gardener, builder and general odd-job man and is very active in his local heart support group.

Ken, 62, had a heart attack when he was 47. Seven years later he had a heart bypass. He is now retired.

Len, 64, had a heart attack when he was 37 and subsequently underwent heart surgery. He and his wife, Linda, a marriage counsellor, started up one of the first UK heart support groups and today counsel people with heart problems and help in the setting up of heart support groups.

Mike is 58, and a former high-flyer in a multinational company. He had a heart attack when he was 50 and a year later had a five-graft bypass. A year after that he had another heart attack. He and his wife now run a heart support group.

Peter, 73, had a quadruple bypass six years ago after he had retired from his job as a civil servant. He is a widower.

Sylvia, 77, started to suffer angina when she was 57 and living in South Africa. She had an aortic aneurysm when she was 69 after moving to the UK. She subsequently had angioplasty. At 73 she had a triple bypass operation and today she lives a full life and is an active member of her local heart support group.

Note: some names have been changed.

Introduction
Heart Disease –
Everyone's Concern

To POETS DOWN THE AGES the heart has been the seat of the emotions. To doctors and scientists it is, more prosaically, a muscular pump that supplies the lungs and the rest of the body with blood. But if you have been given a diagnosis of heart disease your heart is likely to take on a whole new meaning.

The diagnosis of any serious illness tends to bring a mixture of conflicting feelings. Even if you suspected there was a problem with your heart, medical confirmation usually comes as a severe shock. You are likely to be afraid that you will die or, if you live, that your life will be severely limited. The message of this book is that heart disease does not have to be a killer, nor does it have to be crippling; still less does it have to mean the end of your life as you know it.

Medical and surgical treatment have progressed by leaps and bounds and, as you will discover as you read through this book, there are plenty of things you can do to help yourself if you have been diagnosed with heart disease. We'll be looking at all these in later chapters – the first thing to bear in mind is that you are not alone.

A COMMON PROBLEM

Coronary heart disease is the most common serious medical condition affecting people in the Western world. The disease can strike anyone of any age, although it is more common as we grow older. It affects both men and women, rich and poor, black and white. According to the British Heart Foundation, someone, somewhere in the UK has a heart attack every two minutes. This adds up to some 300,000 people each year. Meanwhile, 2 million suffer angina, or pain in the chest, half a million have heart failure and 20,000 others are recovering from heart surgery. American figures tell a similar story. According to the American Heart Association, it is estimated that one in five men and women have some sort of heart disease, adding up to 57 million people. Someone in the US suffers a heart attack every 20 seconds, that's 1,500,000 people a year; 7,120,000 have angina and 350,000 people are diagnosed with it each year. In addition, 2,239,000 Americans are estimated to have atherosclerosis, the hardening and narrowing of the arteries that is the main cause of heart attacks and angina.

Heart disease becomes more common as we get older, partly because the process of atherosclerosis or furring of the arteries is slow and gradual. However, it is not just a disease of the elderly. In fact the condition is often diagnosed when people are in the prime of life with a busy work schedule, children and a myriad other activities and commitments. It is estimated that around half of all middle-aged people have diseased arteries, while the US Framingham Heart Study, one of the most comprehensive pieces of research into heart disease ever undertaken, reveals that 5 per cent of heart attacks occur in the under 40s and 45 per cent in people under 65.

MYTHS AND REALITIES

One of the most tenacious myths about heart disease is that it only affects men. It is only recently that it has begun to be accepted that heart disease is just as much a female problem as it is a male one. In women the disease tends to strike later in life, as before the menopause women have some protection from their female hormones, but they do still suffer from heart disease (see Chapter 9) and by the time a women reaches 65 her risk of developing heart disease is equal to that of a man.

One of the most damaging results of the perception that heart disease mainly affects men is that, in the past especially, the needs of women have often been neglected. There have been several pieces of research showing that heart disease in women is generally less well diagnosed and less well treated and following a heart attack or surgery women have been less likely to be invited to attend or to take up an offer of rehabilitation. Fortunately these days the balance is beginning to be redressed and a growing amount of research is being conducted into the differences and similarities between the sexes.

Another myth about heart disease is that it is solely a disease that affects middle-aged, middle-class, rich businessmen. There is some truth in this to the extent that in poorer parts of the world other diseases tend to get to people first. However, in affluent countries heart disease is just as likely to strike you if you work in a factory as if you are a high-powered executive. Nevertheless, there is some link with your family background, education and earning capacity and much research has been done into this aspect of heart disease. According to a study reported in the *British Medical Journal* in 1997, the key consideration is not so much your job or your income at the point in your life when you are diagnosed with heart disease, but the add-on effect of being exposed to health-damaging environments and influences over the course of your whole lifetime.

Similarly, heart disease has no regard for the colour of your skin, although it has to be said that your racial background may affect your long-term outlook. In the UK South Asians from India, Bangladesh, Pakistan and Sri Lanka are at a particularly high risk of developing heart disease and diabetes (one of the risk factors for heart disease). African Americans – and in the UK people of African-Caribbean background – are more likely to suffer from high blood pressure (a risk of coronary heart disease) and stroke than white people, but in the USA heart disease is slightly more common overall among white people: 7.5 per cent are affected as opposed to 6.9 per cent of black people.

LIVING WITH ANGINA

Unless you discovered you had heart disease when you had a heart attack the chances are high that you sought medical help because of angina, or chest pain. Most people with angina are sent home with a prescription for one of the nitrate drugs – usually glyceryl trinitrate spray which is puffed under your tongue – and expected to get on with it. With treatment most people are able to get on with their lives without undue interference from angina. However, it is worth thinking about the way you live and making adjustments where you can to reduce the number of episodes of angina. One area worth considering is your work commitments.

Not that there is anything wrong with hard work, of course. Work can be a valuable source of self-esteem, and as such be a vital factor in helping you recover and get back to normal. However, if you put work before everything else in your life it is worth having a look at why, and how you might alter things. It may be that you feel unable to say 'No' and therefore tend to take on too much. It could also be that you feel overwhelmed by your work because of poor organization. In this case you may be able to achieve better results for less effort if you learn how to plan and manage your time better.

It is important to keep a balance between work and the rest of your life. Exercise and relaxation are just as important as work and if you have lived a sedentary life until now it is well worth making an extra effort to become more active. You will find more specific advice in Chapters 7 and 12 on what sort of activity to choose and how to keep up your motivation.

It is also a good idea to build in some definite switching-off time into your daily life. Relaxation does not have to mean sitting still doing nothing – activities such as gardening, walking and yoga which involve some physical activity can be equally therapeutic because they allow you to switch off your brain and concentrate on something enjoyable. If you are interested in learning specific relaxation techniques, you will find advice in Chapter 10.

Angina can often be often extremely successfully controlled by medication and management of your lifestyle, but if, despite treatment, angina remains uncontrolled, comes back again or gets worse, you should tell your doctor. He or she may suggest further investigations, a change in medication or a surgical procedure. You will find details about various procedures in Chapter 5. There is no doubt that such procedures can dramatically improve the quality of your life if it is being restricted by severe angina.

GETTING AHEAD OF THE GAME

The good news for anyone diagnosed with heart disease today is that the prospects for the future are brighter than ever before. Over the past few years doctors and scientists have made real strides in understanding and treating the condition and it is true to say that the diagnosis and treatment of heart disease is better than it has ever been.

Improved diagnostic techniques have enabled cardiologists to identify the cause of problems more effectively; surgical techniques such as coronary bypass surgery and angioplasty are now commonplace; while drugs such as ACE inhibitors, cholesterol-lowering drugs, 'clotbusters' and even the humble aspirin have improved the outlook for people with heart disease tremendously.

At the same time, people have taken on the health messages and made changes in their everyday habits to reduce their risk. A huge amount is now known about the various aspects of lifestyle involved in developing heart disease. The latest UK research shows that if you are slim, eat a healthy diet, don't smoke, are moderately active and drink lightly, you have substantially less risk of developing cardiovascular disease. Even if you have already developed heart disease there's a great deal of evidence that paying attention to such factors will help you to recover faster, feel better and fitter and will also help you to avoid other serious diseases such as cancer.

All this new knowledge has had a significant effect on the statistics and today millions of people with heart disease are not just surviving but living healthy, active, enjoyable lives.

The story of heart disease is changing all the time. New discoveries are adding to our understanding of its origins and the factors that can boost the risks. Research has recently revealed, for example, that car exhaust fumes can increase the risk of a heart attack – possibly because carbon monoxide or chemicals in fumes affect the blood's clotting ability. Other new findings have emerged about the role of infection in damaging the arteries. Doctors at St George's Hospital, London, for instance, have discovered that a bacterium that causes the common cold, *Chlamydia pneumoniae*, thrives in atheroma, the sludgy build-up of fats and other debris that furs the arteries. Elsewhere, scientists have discovered that bacteria involved in gum disease may be implicated in the development of atheroma. In both cases treatment with antibiotics could eradicate the infection, so lowering the risk of heart disease. All this increased knowledge helps scientists develop new drugs and more effective treatments and also gives individuals the chance to modify their risk factors.

In the UK the number of men aged between 35 and 74 dying from coronary heart disease fell by 24 per cent and the number of women by 18 per cent in the ten years between 1981 and 1991.

In the USA the improvement is even more striking: the percentage of men aged between 35 and 74 dying of heart disease dropped by 31 per cent and the percentage of women by 30 per cent in the same period. In fact, according to the American Heart Association, over twice as many people survive a heart attack today as did in 1965.

These statistics are especially encouraging because they show what can be achieved by a concerted partnership between doctors and patients. Most of the rest of this book is devoted to just that but before we get on to that let's just look at how the heart works and what can go wrong with it.

CHAPTER 1

MAKING SENSE OF HEART DISEASE

'I kept on getting these pains in my chest when I was going up and down stairs, and in cold, damp weather, a feeling of tightness like bands around my chest, making it difficult to breathe.'

HOWARD, DESCRIBING ANGINA

'When a heart attack hits you, it seems as though a lightning bolt has struck. Few events in life are more frightening. A crushing, breath-robbing pain crashes through your chest. You break into a cold sweat while nausea and a sense of doom overwhelm you.'

ELAINE N. MARIEB, *HUMAN ANATOMY AND PHYSIOLOGY*

WHAT IS CORONARY HEART DISEASE?

The term coronary heart disease (often abbreviated to CHD) is slightly misleading, because it suggests that the heart itself is the main source of the problem. In fact both angina (chest pain) and heart attacks, the two main manifestations of coronary heart disease, are actually caused by narrowing and furring of the **coronary arteries**, the blood vessels which supply the heart muscle with blood and oxygen.

Just as all the tissues and systems of our bodies change with age, our arteries tend to harden and thicken as we get older. Doctors use the term **arteriosclerosis** to describe this general thickening and hardening. Sometimes, for reasons which still aren't entirely clear, the arteries actually become furred and blocked by plaques, fatty deposits of cholesterol and minerals such as calcium which make them hard and brittle. This process is known as **atherosclerosis**. The word *athero* is actually Greek for 'porridge' and describes very accurately the porridge-like sludge that coats the lining of the arteries. When this happens in the coronary arteries it is known as **coronary artery disease**.

Sometimes the plaques crack and bleed, and clots form. This thickens and narrows the arteries still more, leaving ever less room for blood to flow through them, or completely blocks the arteries, causing a heart attack.

THE ORIGINS OF HEART DISEASE

In the past few years doctors and scientists have reached a much more sophisticated understanding of how heart disease develops. In fact, recent studies suggest that the process may stretch back as far as the womb and the first year of life.

Fatty streaks, the first sign of furring of the arteries, have long been known to be present in children's arteries. What researchers still do not understand is why these fatty streaks develop in the first place and what causes them to develop into atheroma, the yellow thickened deposits of fats which are laid down in the arteries.

'In Africa people have fatty streaks but do not develop atheroma,' observes Dr David Newby, lecturer in cardiology at Edinburgh Royal Infirmary. This strongly suggests that atheroma may partly have something to do with aspects of our modern-day environment, such as the food we eat, how active we are, smoking, pollution and other factors in our lifestyle.

THE CHOLESTEROL CONUNDRUM

One of the earliest facts that came to light among doctors and scientists was that people with high cholesterol levels had a higher risk of developing heart disease.

In recent years the experts have come to understand even more about the way cholesterol is involved in heart disease. There are two different types of cholesterol: **low-density lipoprotein (LDL)**, sometimes also known as 'bad' cholesterol, and **high-density lipoprotein (HDL)**, sometimes referred to as 'good' cholesterol. LDL cholesterol is the sort that sticks to the artery walls and raises the risk of heart disease. HDL cholesterol, in contrast, is believed to help clear away LDL cholesterol, so high levels of HDL actually lower the risk to the arteries.

One of the earliest steps in the development of atherosclerosis is when LDL cholesterol is oxidized. Oxidization is the process that causes a cut apple to go brown or butter to go rancid. It is caused by the release of free radicals, rogue molecules which damage cells. When LDL becomes oxidized it causes the accumulation of cells known as foam cells. The formation of foam cells marks the transition from fatty streaks into early atheroma.

OXIDATION AND THE LINING OF THE ARTERIES

Until fairly recently scientists were puzzled by the exact mechanism by which the process of oxidation leads to heart disease. In the past few years a growing amount of research has focused on the part played by the wafer-thin layer of cells lining the heart and blood vessels called the **endothelium**.

The endothelium lubricates blood vessels, allowing blood to flow freely through them. Because it is so thin nutrients and waste products are able to pass easily between the bloodstream and the surrounding tissues. Experts now think that faulty function of the endothelium is a vital early factor in triggering coronary artery disease. This new knowledge has enabled scientists to come up with even more effective treatments for heart disease. Indeed many of the drugs you are likely to have been prescribed if you have heart disease work by acting on the endothelium.

The endothelium may become damaged or injured in various ways: through a virus, high cholesterol, toxic chemicals from, say, cigarettes or pollution, or factors such as high blood pressure.

Scientists are now trying to link what they know about cholesterol with what they have discovered about the endothelium. One of the most convincing theories they have come up with goes something like this. When LDL cholesterol is oxidized it damages neighbouring endothelial cells. In response the endothelium releases agents which cause white blood cells, part of the body's immune defence system, to travel to the damaged area. These white blood cells attach themselves to receptors, special proteins on the surface of the endothelium, rather like keys fitting into a lock. They then burrow beneath the surface of the endothelium where they turn into other cells called macrophages, whose job it is to gobble up invaders and poisons. The macrophages feed greedily on the oxidized LDL until they become so full that they burst, triggering inflammation. It is this inflammation which causes atheroma. 'We still don't know exactly why it happens but it is the beginning of heart disease,' comments Dr Newby.

BLOOD VESSELS AND NITRIC OXIDE

There is another way in which the experts believe endothelium may contribute to the development of heart disease. In normal circumstances the endothelium produces a substance called nitric oxide. This plays a major role both in keeping blood vessels relaxed and open, in preventing clots from forming and in controlling inflammation. If nitric oxide is in short supply the blood vessels go into spasm and blood pressure rises, and high blood pressure is one of the major risk factors for the development of coronary heart disease. How nitric oxide exerts its effects is still unclear, but drugs which release nitric oxide are very useful and in fact that is how the spray or tablets placed under the tongue act to relieve the pain of angina.

THE HORMONAL CONNECTION

Several other important chemicals are secreted by the endothelium. In the past few years a lot of excitement has been generated by the discovery of a powerful hormone called endothelin, which plays a part in causing blood vessels to narrow and in regulating blood pressure. In experiments, animals given drugs designed to counteract the action of endothelin are more likely to survive a heart attack. This paves the way for the future development of new drugs for heart disease.

LEARNING ABOUT THE HEART

One of the most important factors in learning to live with coronary heart disease is being able to make sense of what has happened. Many people find that understanding how their heart works and what can go wrong with it is a step towards coming to grips with what has happened to them and helps them to feel more in control. Clive, for instance, recalls his fascination with a model of the heart he looked at in the cardiac rehabilitation unit: 'I took it apart and looked at it. What really struck me was how small the heart and arteries are. Mine are enlarged because of heart failure. Looking at the models helped me to understand what had happened to me.'

Not everyone is interested in learning about the mechanics of the heart, however, so if you are one of them feel free to skip this section and go on to the next chapter.

HOW THE HEART IS STRUCTURED

The heart is a strong, muscular pump and the toughest organ in the body. As Clive discovered, it is actually surprisingly small, about the size of a man's fist, and weighs just 250–350g (9–12oz). It lies within the ribcage, enclosed in a fibrous sac known as the **pericardium**, with its apex, or lowest point, just below your left nipple. Over the course of an average lifetime the heart expands and contracts some 2500 million times, propelling oxygen and nutrient-rich blood through the circulation to the lungs and the rest of your body.

The heart is divided down the middle by a thick muscular wall called the septum and has four chambers (two on each side). The upper chambers of the heart are called **atria**; the larger, lower chambers are the **ventricles**. The atria receive blood returning to the heart; the ventricles discharge blood back into the circulation and the lungs. Because of the greater work it has to do, the left ventricle is much more powerful than the right, and its walls therefore much thicker.

Blood is pumped through the chambers with the help of four one-way valves, which open and close in response to differences in pressure. The right atrium and the right ventricle are connected to each other by the **tricuspid valve** and the left atrium and left ventricle are connected by the **mitral valve**. The right ventricle is connected to the pulmonary artery by the **pulmonary valve**, while the left ventricle is connected to the aorta by the **aortic valve**. Each heart beat is triggered by electrical impulses produced by the heart's own pacemaker, the **sinoatrial node**. Specialized cells in the heart's muscular walls coordinate to transmit impulses through the muscle fibres, and spread the contraction or heart beat evenly through the chambers of the heart. Your emotions and your hormones can both affect the rate of your heart beat, allowing your body to respond to the various demands, physical or emotional, placed upon it.

THE ARTERIES AND CIRCULATION

There are two main circulations of blood in the body: **pulmonary** (lung) and **systemic** (the rest of the body). The right-hand side of the heart pumps blood though the pulmonary system to oxygenate blood, while the left-hand side pumps blood all the way round the body through the systemic circulation. Equal

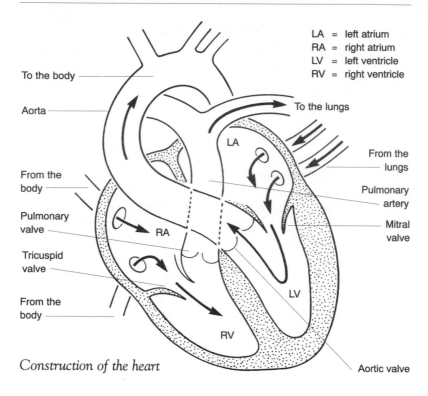

LA = left atrium
RA = right atrium
LV = left ventricle
RV = right ventricle

To the body

Aorta

To the lungs

From the
lungs

From the
body

Pulmonary
artery

Pulmonary
valve

Mitral
valve

Tricuspid
valve

From the
body

Construction of the heart

Aortic valve

volumes of blood, therefore, are flowing in the two circuits at any one time.

To work effectively your heart needs plenty of oxygen and nutrients. These are supplied by the **coronary arteries** – so called because they surround the heart like a crown (from the Latin for crown, *corona*). Things can go wrong with virtually any part of the heart or any aspect of its function, but coronary artery disease is the most common cause of problems.

If the coronary arteries are not functioning efficiently, the body has its own protective mechanism which helps to keep blood flowing to the heart. This is known as the **collateral circulation**. We all have rudimentary collateral blood vessels, small arteries which connect larger arteries or join different segments of the same artery. Normally these vessels remain small and closed, but they can grow and enlarge to provide a detour around a blocked artery, creating an alternative route for blood to flow to the heart. In this way the body helps to protect itself against heart attack.

So, what can go wrong?

HEART ATTACK

For two-thirds of men the first clue that there is anything wrong with their heart is having a heart attack. It can be terrifying, as the quotes at the beginning of this chapter reveal. However, the pain is not always so overwhelming, as Jim, who had a mild attack, recalls: 'I felt a pain in my left arm when I was running. It didn't cross my mind that it was anything to do with my heart. My doctor thought it was probably a trapped nerve. It was only when he sent me for tests that it was found I'd had a heart attack.' Ken's experience was different again: 'Imagine a hand squeezing very rapidly. It wasn't so much painful as a feeling that I wanted it to stop because I didn't know what it was. I felt I couldn't sit still. I wanted to get in a different position. I even remember thinking if I could climb up the wall it might help. I was sweating and I felt sick and I was a pasty colour.'

WHAT CAUSES A HEART ATTACK?

A heart attack, or **myocardial infarction** to use the medical term, happens when the blood supply to a part of the heart muscle, or myocardium, is interrupted or stops. This interruption to the blood flow is usually the result of a blockage caused by a blood clot or thrombosis which has formed on the plaque due to atherosclerosis.

Rarely, a heart attack can also be caused by spasm of a coronary artery. When this happens the artery narrows, reducing or stopping the blood flow to the heart. It is not known exactly why the arteries go into spasm, but healthy blood vessels, not only those furred by atherosclerosis, can go into spasm.

Whatever the underlying mechanism, when the heart muscle cells are deprived of blood, they become starved of oxygen and die. But the heart is amazingly resilient, and tough scar tissue soon forms in the area that was deprived of blood, while the rest of the heart takes over the work that was previously done by the damaged part.

In the past it was thought that it was only lack of oxygen in itself which caused the cells to die, but it has now been discovered that the story is more complicated. When blood flows back into the part of the heart which has been starved of blood, white blood cells produced by the immune system and other inflammatory cells begin to accumulate in the area. These cells release cytokines, chemical messengers, which in turn trigger a torrent of free radicals, harmful molecules that destroy cells. It is now thought that the damage to the heart is worsened by this flood of free radicals, aggravating the depression of the action of the heart and causing fatal damage to its tissue.

How severe a heart attack is depends on which part of the heart is deprived of oxygen and how much tissue dies. Sometimes the damage is so severe that the heart stops beating altogether – this is **cardiac arrest**. However, most people who die as a result of a heart attack do so because the attack throws the heart's pumping mechanism out of sync, upsetting its rhythm.

VENTRICULAR FIBRILLATION

There are many different causes to a disturbance in the heart's rhythm, but the type that occurs after a heart attack is called **ventricular fibrillation**. Instead of beating regularly, the heart begins to beat abnormally rapidly and chaotically and starts to quiver.

Left untreated, ventricular fibrillation is usually fatal. However, if you are in hospital or an ambulance when ventricular fibrillation sets in, the heart's rhythm can be restored by using a device called a **defibrillator**. This delivers an electric charge which stimulates the heart to resume its normal beat. The use of defibrillation since the 1960s, together with the more recent introduction of 'clotbusting' drugs to dissolve clots and restore blood flow, is one of the reasons why so many more people survive heart attacks today than did 30 years ago.

Ventricular fibrillation is most common in the first hour after a heart attack and becomes less of a risk over the following six hours, which is why it is so crucial to get medical help immediately if you suspect you or someone close to you is having a heart attack.

IS IT A HEART ATTACK?

According to some estimates half of all the people who die from a heart attack do so because they did not seek medical help soon enough. Many people delay seeking help because they attribute their symptoms to angina or indigestion and try to treat them themselves. Some people are so afraid of the possibility of a heart attack that they refuse to acknowledge even to themselves that they are having one. Others, even those who have had a heart attack before, are afraid of bothering the doctor in case it turns out to be a false alarm.

Research suggests that people tend to put off seeking help longer if there is someone else present, perhaps because they feel they should underplay their symptoms, be brave or fear looking foolish. If you do suspect a heart attack there is no point in being stoical. It's important that both you and your nearest and dearest recognize the symptoms of a heart attack and know what to do and when to seek help.

SYMPTOMS OF A HEART ATTACK

If you experience any of the following, get medical help straight away:

- A persistent, crushing, burning pain in the centre of the chest that lasts for more than a few minutes or goes away and then comes back
- A pain that seems to 'wrap' itself around your body
- Pain that spreads to your shoulders, neck or arms. Pain may also be felt in the throat, jaw, back or abdomen
- Pain that does not go away with rest
- Chest discomfort with feelings of weakness, dizziness, light-headedness or faintness, chill, sweating, nausea, vomiting or breathlessness

As well as these physical symptoms many people experience an intangible feeling of unease. According to the *Yale Heart Book* this can range from a 'sense of impending doom' to a feeling that 'something isn't quite right'.

ACTION

Because of the danger of cardiac arrest both during a heart attack and in people who have coronary heart disease, it's a very good idea to have an action plan. This should include a knowledge of **cardiopulmonary resuscitation (CPR)** so that anyone who is with you when you have a heart attack can keep the blood flowing to the heart and brain in an emergency. Learning the technique of CPR can literally be lifesaving. When given immediately to someone in cardiac arrest their chance of survival is 25–30 per cent. When it is delayed until the emergency services arrive the chance of survival drops to 5 per cent. Irreversible brain damage occurs within 4–6 minutes of having a cardiac arrest.

The technique of CPR is easily learnt. In the UK the British Heart Foundation's Heartstart UK initiative has been set up to train people in emergency support and resuscitation techniques. In the US contact the American Heart Association. For advice on what to do in an emergency, see Appendix 1.

ANGINA

The other common way in which coronary heart disease makes itself felt is angina, or **angina pectoris**, as doctors call it, which simply means 'pain in the chest'. This is especially true of women – for 56 per cent of women angina is the first clue that they have heart disease. Gill, 53, recalls: 'There was nothing very definite: just feeling unusual, breathless, with a very slight pain in my chest, always on exertion. On one occasion my husband and I were making love and I got the same feeling. He asked, "What's the matter?" and I said, "I feel strange." We stopped and the feeling went away. It kept happening on and off.'

WHAT ANGINA FEELS LIKE

The pain of angina can vary in severity from a slight twinge to a severe, crushing pain. The pain is usually centred in the chest, although it may radiate out to the neck, shoulder, arm or lower jaw. Occasionally the pain is felt in these areas alone and not in the chest. It usually comes on gradually and lasts for several minutes and is often accompanied by breathlessness.

Carolyn recalls her first experience of angina: 'We went away for a long weekend to Stratford-upon-Avon. Two of the evenings were very damp and cold and I started getting a tightness in my throat and couldn't catch my breath properly. In the morning after a rest it was OK. The next day we decided to go to Warwick Castle. We parked the car but I hadn't got half way up the hill when I felt pain in both arms and my ribs and a tightening in my chest. My husband put it down to anxiety but I knew deep down that something physical was wrong. I went to the doctor who in turn sent me to see a specialist and he diagnosed angina.'

Clive describes angina as 'a somewhat dull pain with tightening of the chest and a feeling of breathlessness, but it's never really stopped me or made me double up'.

CAUSES OF ANGINA

The symptoms of angina are caused by a phenomenon known as **myocardial ischaemia**. 'Ischaemia' is the medical term for lack of blood supply and 'myocardial' refers to the myocardium or heart muscle. In myocardial ischaemia narrowing and furring of the coronary arteries prevents sufficient oxygen-rich blood reaching the heart muscle. The circulation to your heart may be sufficient to meet most everyday needs but falls short if your heart's needs increase as a result of extra physical exertion such as climbing upstairs, a game of tennis, running for a bus or having sex.

Angina can also be brought on by emotional stress. This is because when the body perceives any sort of extra demand, be it emotional or physical, it prepares to deal with it either by facing it or by running away from it. This is the so-called 'fight or flight' reaction involved in stress, and either option sends messages to your body to prepare for action. Angina is also more common after a meal or in cold weather.

Rarely, angina can be caused by the arteries going into spasm rather than atherosclerosis, as Dr David Newby explains: 'There are three or four types which are brought on by spasm of the arteries. These may be linked to other conditions involving spasm of the blood vessels such as migraine, Raynaud's syndrome (in which circulation to the hands and feet is constricted) and can be associated in some cases with indigestion. You can, of course, have atheroma on top of spasm.'

STABLE AND UNSTABLE ANGINA

There are two types of angina. The sort known as **stable angina** is predictable. People with it can often pinpoint exactly how far they have to walk, for instance, before a bout begins. Clive says: 'I would develop a shocking pain like a knife blade sticking in my upper arm with shortness of breath which would come on after I'd been walking a couple of hundred yards and I'd have to stop and wait for it to go away before I carried on walking.'

Unstable angina is, as its name suggests, unpredictable. Pain begins to strike more often or is present even when you are resting. If your angina has previously been stable but becomes unstable you should report it to your doctor as it can sometimes be a sign of an impending heart attack.

The key clue that chest pain is caused by angina rather than by a heart attack is that angina disappears once you stop doing whatever it was that triggered it and rest. Some people imagine that angina is a 'mini heart attack' but this in fact is not the case. In a heart attack, some of the heart's muscle cells actually die. In angina, despite the temporary lack of oxygen, the muscle cells remain alive and continue to function.

This understanding is important because research shows that people with angina sometimes wrongly believe that their heart is weak and that they should not do too much. This often creates a vicious circle in which the less you do the less you are able to do, until your life is severely limited. There is evidence to suggest that the exact opposite is true: by gradually becoming more active you can increase the capacity of your heart to deal with extra demands and angina frequently becomes less of a problem. You'll find more advice on dealing with angina in Chapter 2.

SILENT ISCHAEMIA

The presence of obvious symptoms of heart disease such as angina or a heart attack gives you the opportunity to seek diagnosis and treatment, but for many people heart disease creeps up stealthily. Although the arteries are narrowed and the heart muscle starved of oxygen they experience no warnings. Some people even have tiny heart attacks without being aware of the fact. Such silent heart attacks may only show up later during hospital tests when a part of the heart is discovered to be damaged.

The medical term for this symptomless oyxgen starvation is **silent ischaemia** (ischaemia being the medical word for lack of blood supply). The American Heart Association estimates that as many as three to four million Americans may be affected by silent ischaemia. There are no similar British figures, but according to Belinda Linden, nurse adviser at the British Heart Foundation: 'About 40 per cent of people who undergo a treadmill test may have silent ischaemia. It is especially likely to affect people with diabetes, older people and women.'

No one knows exactly why some people have silent ischaemia but there are hints that those with it may have abnormal pain mechanisms. 'Diabetes can affect the nerves, so people with it may not feel heart pain, while in older people pain sensations may be lost because of degenerative changes in their nerves,' explains Dr David Newby.

The danger of silent ischaemia, of course, is that you are not in a position to stop doing any activity which triggers it, and are less likely to be diagnosed with heart disease or receive treatment and so are more at risk of having an unexpected heart attack. Some people learn they have a problem by chance during a routine health check or screening (the condition is diagnosed by an exercise test – see page 35).

ATYPICAL SYMPTOMS

Sometimes people with heart disease do have symptoms but fail to identify them as being connected to their heart. The atypical symptoms may include pain in the jaw, heaviness in the left arm and sometimes pain in the shoulder or back, or niggling 'indigestion' that goes on over several weeks, especially when these are associated with exercise plus a vague feeling of unease that you cannot quite put a finger on. 'Because diabetes causes loss of sensation,' says Dr David Newby, 'people with it may present with vomiting and a feeling of vague unwellness or flu and it is only when you do an ECG that you realize they have had a heart attack.'

Individual sensations vary widely. Peter comments: 'At the beginning it felt like indigestion and things like belching relieved it.' Ken recalls: 'During the six months before I had the heart attack I suffered dizzy spells and I kept collapsing, my legs would just cave in under me. People at work thought I was messing about. I went to the doctor who said, "It's just one of those things." Eventually I collapsed again at work one day and someone called an ambulance. I spent the weekend in hospital but they couldn't find anything wrong. They wrote a letter to the doctor which said, "Definitely not heart". Six weeks later I had a heart attack.'

Carolyn says: 'I noticed that I would get a bit out of breath if I walked up a hill, but I put it down to being unfit.' It was only when she experienced a severe reaction to a prescribed migraine drug that heart disease was suspected: 'I developed really severe chest pains that went on for about 20 minutes. My husband phoned the doctor who said it's usually only older people who get a reaction like this. I was sent to the hospital who did an ECG. That was abnormal. They did another one about half an hour later and that was abnormal too, so they took me in and I ended up in hospital for three days. They did tests and took blood samples and said I hadn't had a heart attack but that marked the start of my angina.'

The coronary arteries are not the only ones where atheroma can develop. Cramp-like pain in the calves or thighs when walking or exercising but which disappears after a few moments' rest may be a warning that the arteries in the legs have become narrowed or furred up. This is called **intermittent claudication**. John remembers: 'I had been getting cramps in my legs whenever I exercised. I didn't think too much of it but it didn't go away and started to get worse. At the time I was in the Territorial Army. We had to do a 30km route march for a local disabled school and I had the ignominy of dropping out of the squad. Eventually things became so bad I could barely keep up with my three-year-old son.' Although not directly related to the heart, intermittent claudication may indicate that atheroma is building up elsewhere; John later suffered a silent heart attack.

Although it is easy to be wise after the event, symptoms can be misleading, as Belinda Linden, nurse adviser with the British Heart Foundation points out: 'Such symptoms are very difficult to interpret because they are so varied. However, if people do experience them or anything else they are worried about it is worth seeing the doctor, especially where someone has experienced other problems previously, such as sweating or nausea linked to exertion or cold weather. They may just be the clue that completes the picture.'

PALPITATIONS AND ARRHYTHMIAS – DISTURBANCES OF HEART RHYTHM

Normally the heart beats at a rate of between 50 and 100 beats a minute, depending on what we are doing. We all experience variations in heart rhythm as we go about our everyday lives – our heart beats faster, for example, when we exercise, if we are excited or under stress, and slows down when we are relaxed or sleeping.

Sometimes we become aware of our heart beating – especially if it seems to be going too fast. This is known as **palpitation** and is usually quite harmless. Palpitations are often brought on by feeling nervous or angry, by exercise, a raised temperature, a stomach upset, alcohol or even over-the-counter cold cures. However, if you have had a heart attack these normal palpitations may cause great anxiety because you may fear you are having another heart attack.

People with coronary heart disease, atherosclerosis, high blood pressure and other changes in the blood vessels are prone to more marked variations in rhythm (called **arrhythmias**). This is because scarring or abnormal tissue deposits may disturb the electrical signalling system within the heart's own pacemaker, the sinoatrial node. This may cause the heart's cells to fire abnormally or create patches of electrically inert tissue, which in turn can cause the heart to beat abnormally fast (the medical term is **tachycardia**) or abnormally slowly (**bradycardia**).

We have already seen that a heart attack may set the ventricles beating fast and irregularly (**ventricular fibrillation**). Another important and common type of tachycardia is known as **atrial fibrillation**. In this type of arrhythmia the atria (the upper chambers of the heart) beat extremely rapidly – the rate can reach 400 beats a minute. The AV node, which sends impulses from the atria to the ventricles, cannot cope with this and therefore sends only a selection of the impulses to the ventricles. As a result the ventricles beat quickly (say 180 beats a minute) and irregularly. Although the palpitations of atrial fibrillation can feel very unpleasant they are not immediately dangerous.

Fortunately most palpitations are a nuisance rather than life-threatening and many can be cured by avoiding trigger factors such as alcohol or over-the-counter cold remedies. More serious arrhythmias may need to be treated with special drugs; you will find more details on these in Chapter 4. Alternatively, the doctor may suggest implanting a pacemaker or another procedure to regularize the heart's rhythm.

VALVE PROBLEMS AND HEART FAILURE

When a large part of the heart muscle dies in a single heart attack, or if you have several heart attacks in succession so that the heart does not have time to recover, the muscles may become so weakened they can no longer pump properly. This is known as heart failure.

A heart attack can also weaken the heart's valves, causing them to become leaky (the medical term is **incompetent** or **regurgitant**). This is very rare, and problems with the valves are more usually a result of rheumatic fever during childhood, inborn valve defects or infection. When valves are diseased they may become narrowed or **stenosed**, just like blood vessels. 'Sometimes the muscle cells in the heart's valves die in a heart attack and when this happens the valve starts flopping. This can also happen in the septum, the membrane that divides the two parts of the heart,' explains Dr David Newby.

Such problems with the valves also strain the heart because as well as pumping the blood forward as it normally does the blood also goes backwards through the valves. Leakage from the mitral and aortic valves on the left side of the heart cause the left ventricle to thicken and enlarge to cope with the extra work it has to do. Eventually, under the strain, the left ventricle fails and this leads to breathlessness. The back pressure on the lungs in turn makes extra work for the right ventricle which may not be able to cope. When this happens the right ventricle fails, causing fluid retention and swelling in the legs, ankles and abdomen.

STROKE

Coronary heart disease may also push up your risk of experiencing certain types of **stroke** (in the US this is sometimes called a **brain attack**). Like a heart attack, a stroke happens when one of the blood vessels supplying the brain with oxygen and nutrients bursts or becomes clogged by a blood clot or particle of other material, depriving that area of the brain of blood. As a result the deprived cells die and the part of the body controlled by that area of brain cells is unable to work, causing perhaps loss of speech or the inability to move a hand or arm.

CHAPTER 2

DISCOVERING YOU HAVE HEART DISEASE

'It is hard to describe the feelings – I felt unusual, breathless with a very slight pain in my chest always on exertion.'

GILL

'The problem is, if you get a pain in your chest you tend to pass it off as indigestion. If you get a tingle down your arm you dismiss it. I was tired and irritable for months before my heart attack.'

MIKE

'Heart disease isn't a sudden thing; it creeps up on you. There's nothing on the outside, no lump or anything to show you are ill.'

LINDA

GETTING A DIAGNOSIS

If you have had a heart attack or been admitted into hospital for heart surgery there is little doubt that you have heart disease. However, not everyone has such a clear-cut indication of problems. If you suspect there might be something wrong with your heart your first step should be to make an appointment with your family doctor.

In the UK the family doctor is the means by which you can gain access to the services of the NHS. He or she is there to make an initial diagnosis, answer questions, make referrals to a specialist for further tests and help you find other services such as counselling or physiotherapy. An increasing number of doctors run their own groups for heart patients. Many surgeries also run stop smoking groups, stress management groups and groups for people who are trying to lose weight.

DIAGNOSTIC DILEMMAS

Unfortunately it isn't always easy to get a diagnosis, especially if your symptoms are vague, untypical or occur at an age when you would not normally expect to have a heart attack. Len was just 33 when he experienced a heart attack. His wife, Linda, recalls: 'We were playing cards with friends when he got terrible pain across his chest that wouldn't go away. He went to the doctor and was seen by a locum who said, "I don't like what I hear." When he went back to see our own doctor, however, he was told: "It's a muscle spasm." All the ECGs were clear, but he wasn't given a stress test.'

Len continued to feel unwell with pains in his chest. Linda says: 'Some time later Len took his car for a service. It was a bitterly cold day and he couldn't walk up the hill because of the pain in his chest. He said, "I've just taken the car for a service and it cost me £150. I can do the same for my body." He went to the doctor and said, "I don't care what you say, I want to see a specialist." He was referred to a cardiologist who gave Len a stress test. After two minutes he said, "I can see what's wrong." '

Linda's advice is: 'No one knows your body like you do. Don't be fobbed off – even if you waste someone's time it's not so awful.' Women in particular may sometimes find that it takes longer to be diagnosed, partly because doctors may be less likely to be looking for heart disease in women than they are in men, as we shall see in Chapter 9.

Gill backs this up: 'The most important thing is to persevere. Even though my doctor wasn't convinced there was anything wrong I was sure something was the matter. In fact, I was on my way to the doctor's when I passed out running for the bus. Later my doctor said, "You knew didn't you? I might not have picked it up if you hadn't passed out." '

Clive had silent ischaemia and only discovered he had a problem with his heart when he went for a routine check-up as part of a research study: 'I had to go to a hospital once a year for a mental and physical check-up. On this occasion they gave me a brown envelope and told me to go and see my family doctor. He took my blood pressure and told me there was nothing to worry about, although he asked me to come back once a month to have my blood pressure taken.

A few weeks later at a Christmas party the ceiling suddenly started going round and I began to sweat. I felt so peculiar I lay down on the settee. My friends thought I was drunk but luckily there were some nurses there who realized it was more serious than that and called an ambulance.' Clive was having a heart attack and it was discovered he had three blocked coronary arteries. He ended up staying in hospital for three weeks and subsequently had a heart bypass.

Clive still feels angry about about what he perceives as his doctor's lack of interest: 'The hospital has been brilliant but my family doctor hasn't. First of all he ignored the information in the brown envelope. Then after my heart attack he said: "These things happen. I made a mistake." '

HELPING YOUR DOCTOR HELP YOU

Doctors are not magicians and it can sometimes be difficult for them to interpret symptoms, especially if, as they often do, they include rather vague complaints such as 'feeling peculiar' or 'feeling uneasy'. Even if you do have the classic symptom of chest pain it is not always easy for the doctor to identify the cause, as Dr David Newby points out: 'Much depends on the personality of the patient: sometimes people don't complain at all even though they have quite severe symptoms, others notice every twinge. Chest pain can have a whole range of different causes. If you get a patient complaining of it you have to try to quantify the risk. It is all to do with the level of suspicion. If the patient complains of classic symptoms it's easy, but unfortunately people sometimes come saying I've had too much to eat and complain of a tiny, vague pain. While in some people the only sign of angina is very bad gum ache. The test to prove if it is heart disease is angiography (see below) but that in itself can cause problems so we don't do it lightly.'

Of course, no doctor can predict definitively that a patient is going to have a heart attack, and no one can blame a doctor who makes an honest mistake. If you feel that your doctor has taken the trouble to listen to you and talk you through the various alternatives you are likely to feel more satisfied than if you feel the doctor has been dismissive as he sadly was in Clive's case –

even if his or her diagnosis does prove ultimately to be wrong.

Of course, some people do not want to know too much about their condition and are quite happy to leave everything to the doctor. However many people with heart disease have a need for clear, understandable information. If you are not satisfied with the way your doctor deals with you and talking it over does not help, Dr David Newby suggests asking for a second opinion. On your part you can help your doctor by trying to be as specific as you can about your symptoms and by keeping an accurate note of where and when you experience them and how long they last.

DIAGNOSTIC TESTS

A huge number of diagnostic tests are available for detecting heart disease. The following are the most common. They may be used to diagnose heart disease or to assess your condition if you already have heart disease. They are listed in alphabetical order, not order of importance.

ANGIOGRAPHY (CARDIAC CATHETERIZATION)

The 'gold standard' of diagnosis is the special type of X-ray called an **angiogram**. It is done under local anaesthetic and these days is one of the most common 'advanced' diagnostic tests performed. A fine tube (catheter) is introduced into an artery in your forearm or groin. This is passed along the body's arteries until it reaches the coronary arteries. A dye is then injected which shows up on an X-ray. This shows where and by how much the arteries are narrowed. It may be used if you go complaining of chest pain, to define the function of the heart and check on narrowing or leaking of the heart valves. It is also used if angioplasty or coronary artery surgery is being considered. John described angiography as 'a weird sensation like a hot flush. It feels like you're going to wet yourself.'

BLOOD TESTS

A blood test may be done to measure the amount of cholesterol and other blood constituents. After a heart attack or suspected heart attack blood tests can be done which measure enzymes released into the blood stream by damaged heart muscle. This helps confirm diagnosis of a heart attack and provides some indication of the extent of damage to the heart muscle.

CHEST X-RAY

Another very simple and common test that may be done is to look at the size and shape of your heart and to look for signs of congestion in the lungs which could indicate heart failure. It can also show calcium deposits which might indicate scarring or blockages in the arteries and swelling of the aorta, the main blood vessel leaving the heart, which might be a sign of a weakness in the wall of the aorta.

ECHOCARDIOGRAM

This is an ultrasound scan of the heart. A small probe or transducer is passed over your chest to produce different views of your heart as it beats. This allows the doctor to view the heart's structure and pumping action. When combined with a Doppler scan (which records changes in the frequency of sound waves) it can also measure blood flow through the heart valves and within the heart's chambers. It is also possible to do three-dimensional echocardiograms.

ELECTROCARDIOGRAM (ECG), TREADMILL TEST OR STRESS TEST

One of the simplest and most routine tests used to help diagnose heart disease. A number of electrodes are attached to your chest and limbs so as to record the electrical activity of your heart. This is recorded on a print-out. An ECG is often referred to as a **stress test**. The test may be done when you are resting (**a resting ECG**) or when you are active, for example walking on a treadmill or pedalling a stationary bicycle, in which case it is called an **exercise stress test**. It can detect changes which may result from reduced blood supply (ischaemia) and also irregularities of heart rhythm. For some reason stress tests seem to be less accurate in women without symptoms than men without symptoms. An ECG also shows the changes linked to healing after a heart attack and may be done before you leave hospital after a heart attack or shortly after returning home.

HOLTER/AMUBULATOR MONITORING

This is a 24-hour ECG that monitors your heart's activity over the course of a complete day. This is recorded on magnetic tape and then analysed by computer. It provides useful information about abnormalities of heart rhythm.

THALLIUM SCAN

A small amount of radioactive substance (usually no longer thallium but the name has stuck) is injected into the blood. A special camera is then used to take a series of photographs to show which parts of the heart muscle are deprived of blood. When a thallium scan is combined with a stress test (or, if exercise would be difficult, you may be given a drug that simulates exercise) it can define the extent of damage and areas of the heart getting insufficient blood. The whole thing takes around 20–45 minutes. Following a period of rest a set of photos showing your heart at rest will be taken and in some cases a third set of photos is taken 24 hours later.

Gill recalls: 'They give you this stuff and put you on a bike and then you have to cycle to get it through your body. I had the most awful chest pains. It takes a very long time and then takes an hour for the computer to collate. Because I was a private patient the doctor let me sit with him. My heart should have been bright green. As it was there was only one speck of green in the middle.'

WHAT NEXT?

Once your doctor has reached a diagnosis he or she may decide to prescribe drug treatment for the relief of angina, drugs to lower your blood pressure and so on. Alternatively, you may be referred to a cardiologist, a doctor who specializes in heart problems, for further diagnostic tests and/or treatment. You will find details of these in subsequent chapters.

COMING TO TERMS WITH HEART DISEASE

IMMEDIATE REACTIONS

If you have been told you have heart disease both you and those around you may feel very frightened, especially if diagnosis was sudden or unexpected. Linda recalls: 'The heart evokes a lot of emotion. When Len was told he needed surgery we walked out in silence holding each other's hands. I thought I ought to be saying comforting things but I couldn't think of anything to say.

'After he had been admitted, I walked away. Had it been any other type of surgery I wouldn't have been so frightened. It was February and the stores were full of Valentines all with hearts on them. It was a visible reminder of what Len was going through. When I returned to the hospital I was so terrified my legs dragged. I knew the surgeon was going to come towards me and say, "I'm sorry, Mrs Shane..." Of course he didn't. Len was terrified too. He put everything in order.'

INTIMATIONS OF MORTALITY

Even if you haven't had a full-blown heart attack, being told that you have heart disease is one of the most distressing pieces of news you are ever likely to have to face. Being forced to confront your own mortality can cause you to re-evaluate every aspect of your life.

In fact many people with the condition say afterwards that having a heart attack or learning they had heart disease was a significant turning point in their lives.

The realization that you have a potentially fatal condition can help you to focus on what is important to you in life in a way that nothing else does. There often follows a period of soul-searching during which you take a close look at your life and think about the way you want to live it in the future. The idea that heart disease can be an opportunity for change and growth is backed by a telling piece of Scandinavian research carried out in 1988. A third of those interviewed looking back a year after a heart attack reported that their quality of life was actually better than it had been before.

Unfortunately by no means everyone who has had a heart attack experiences such a positive outcome. A third of people in the same study said that their quality of life had remained unchanged and a third thought their life was poorer than it was before their heart attack. Although there has been very little specific research into people who have angina, heart failure or who have had heart surgery, what little there is suggests that their experiences may be similar.

WILL I EVER GET BACK TO NORMAL?

Studies are now being carried out looking at the best ways of alleviating the anxiety and unhappiness of the third of people whose quality of life is diminished by having heart disease. If you have just been diagnosed you will want to know what you can do now to regain your sense of well-being so you can count yourself among the first group: those whose lives change for the better.

British cardiac rehabilitation expert, Professor Bob Lewin, argues that people who have had a heart attack – and the same could apply equally well to anyone suffering from heart disease generally – have several well-defined needs. These include the need for clear, understandable, honest facts about their condition and outlook; a clear idea of when they can resume their normal activities; when and if they should return to work; how much activity is safe and which exercises are helpful or harmful; knowledge of what to do to prevent a heart attack and what to do in case of an emergency.

An open, honest discussion with your own doctor is the best way to get advice on the specific details of your particular condition and how to deal with it. As far as the other needs are concerned, you can go a long way to meeting them yourself. One of the worst things about any serious or chronic illness is that it can make you feel out of control of your own life. Taking the reins into your own hands by doing what you can to become healthy will help restore your sense of control over your own destiny.

THE ROAD TO RECOVERY

Following a diagnosis of heart disease, a heart attack or heart surgery it often takes some time before you start living life to the full again. Just how long will vary depending on your condition. If you have had a heart attack or heart surgery you will have spent a period in hospital. You will need time to recover physically and this may well take several months. You will also need emotional recovery time. If you were admitted to hospital as an emergency you are likely to be feeling shaken and you may need a longer period to come to terms with what has happened to you than someone whose admission was planned.

It takes time to adjust to the knowledge that you have coronary heart disease. You are likely to have to get used to taking regular medication for angina or high blood pressure, for example.

You may have been advised that you need an operation, such as a coronary bypass or angioplasty and put on a waiting list. You will find more details of what these involve and how you can cope with them in the next two chapters.

Professor Lewin points out that one of the main reasons it can be so difficult to come to terms with heart disease is that – unlike many other unfortunate events that happen in life, such as being involved in an accident or being made redundant – a diagnosis of heart disease can't be dismissed as a one-off piece of bad luck that is unlikely ever to strike again. From now on you have to live with the constant reality that you have a long-term health problem.

You may also have practical worries about whether you will be able to continue working, how you will manage to pay the bills if you have to stop and the effect this will have on your standard of living. Taking some time to think constructively about such concerns, talking to the relevant people and setting in motion some practical plans rather than just worrying will go a long way to alleviate such anxieties. You'll find some suggestions, together with details of how other people have coped, in Chapter 11.

NEGATIVE THINKING

By far the greatest barrier to adjusting to a diagnosis of heart disease, according to Professor Lewin, is thinking negatively about the condition. Myths and half-truths about heart disease abound. These may be fuelled by gossip about people who 'just dropped dead of a heart attack with no warning' and lurid stories in the media about famous people who died of a 'massive heart attack'. (In fact, people who die suddenly are most often victims of sudden cardiac arrest, when the heart stops beating, rather than a 'massive heart attack'.)

Professor Lewin comments that people are often (wrongly) convinced that a heart attack will strike them dead at any moment. They frequently – and again wrongly – blame themselves for having brought their condition on themselves by being a worrier, working too hard or being stressed.

Not surprisingly, seeing your disease in such a light is likely to make you miserable and anxious because it renders you powerless to do anything about it. Unfortunately doctors sometimes unintentionally reinforce negative views of heart disease because they often talk a different language from lay people. Dr Chris

Isles, a physician at Dumfries Infirmary in Scotland who has a special interest in heart disease, says: 'When a cardiologist says "Your heart is weak" he means that, seen on an echocardiogram, the blood the heart expels is less than it should be. What the patient interprets by this is that their heart has worn out and they are going to die.' (Whereas, as we saw in the previous chapter, the heart is an extremely tough organ that even when damaged repairs itself.)

It is always much easier to deal with reality than it is with vague fears based on what you think is true. For this reason it is important to make sure you understand exactly what your doctor is telling you by asking for clarification of any terms that you have not understood and asking him or her to explain the practical implications of any statements made about your condition.

LEARNING TO THINK MORE POSITIVELY

Professor Lewin argues that replacing the mistaken beliefs that many people have about heart disease – 'cardiac misconceptions' as he calls them – with more realistic facts is one of the most significant ways in which you can help yourself recover.

'Few people believe which were the real risk factors responsible for their getting heart disease. They say things like, "I might have smoked, but it was the stress that got me." This is extremely damaging because it leads people to rest as much as possible. That is the worst thing you can do, because the less you do the more likely you are to experience angina and the more likely you are to become depressed,' he observes.

He believes that everyone who has had a diagnosis of heart disease should be given accurate information about their condition, its outlook and the changes they need to make, preferably in a structured counselling session. 'Just talking about feelings is of absolutely no benefit,' he says. 'People need to rid themselves of misconceptions or be given some way of coping with them.'

Most people will not have such a session, but there are things you can do to help yourself develop a more positive way of thinking. First of all it's worth reminding yourself that heart disease is a *disease* and not a sign that your body has worn out – even when the arteries are diseased the body has its own safety mechanism in the form of the collateral circulation described in

Chapter 1. In the vast majority of cases the heart heals rapidly, even after a heart attack.

Secondly, you should be aware that these days a diagnosis of heart disease is far from being an automatic death sentence. The fact that you now are under medical surveillance means that any problems are likely to be picked up and dealt with before they become life threatening.

Finally, it pays to bear in mind that by far the biggest causes of heart disease are not stress, worry and hard work but identifiable factors such as smoking, high cholesterol, lack of activity and so on, and that these are things you can do something about.

If you are having difficulty convincing yourself of any of this, it may be helpful to take some steps to improve your knowledge by making a special appointment with your doctor or calling a cardiac helpline such as the ones run by various hospitals or heart charities. You could also check out a few of the books on heart disease. If you decide to seek information from medical books from a library, however, make sure that the ones you choose are up to date. Knowledge and treatment is changing all the time and books written even five years ago may be a source of wrong or mis-leading information which can make you unnecessarily gloomy.

ANGINA MANAGEMENT PROGRAMMES

Research shows that a combination of techniques used in pain management together with cognitive behavioural psychology methods in which people are encouraged to change the way they think about angina and set themselves progressive goals to increase activity and control pain can be successful in helping angina sufferers live more normal lives.

In one or two areas of the UK these ideas and techniques form the basis of an Angina Management Programme used by psychologists working with cardiologists. Such a programme typically includes looking at mistaken beliefs that may increase pain and limit activity, learning self-help ways of coping with angina such as relaxation and breathing, a programme of gentle exercise to be done at home, yoga and stress-management techniques designed to help people face stressful situations that normally bring on an attack of chest pain.

'People with heart disease and their families often think angina is like a mini-heart attack,' explains Dr Nicola Stuckey, 'and think that they should avoid doing things. As a result they set up a cycle of fear and avoidance.' Dr Stuckey runs an Angina Management Programme at the British Heart Foundation's Rehabilitation Research Unit at the Astley Ainsley Hospital in Edinburgh, Scotland. The programme consists of 13 half-day sessions held over ten weeks.

Participants are encouraged to keep an Angina Diary in which they record how often and how severely they experience symptoms and how long bouts last. They are also asked to pinpoint activities which they have cut down or stopped doing because of angina or fatigue such as DIY, gardening, dancing, fishing, bowls and going out with friends, or sometimes more solitary activities like reading, writing and knitting. The next step is for participants to set themselves mini-goals, so they gradually start doing more and build up the number of activities and time spent doing them. 'The main factor is that all the activity is done at the patient's own pace so they are in control,' observes Dr Stuckey.

By the time they have been through the programme most people find they are able to do more and experience fewer symptoms. A large number also find that doing a breathing or rapid relaxation technique enables them to give up using their aerosol spray, while a few are so much better able to cope that they are able to come off the waiting list for surgery altogether. Others find that the programme makes symptoms more bearable during their wait for an operation. Such a programme can also be extremely helpful if, for any reason, the doctor decides that you are not suitable for or would not benefit from surgery.

Angina management programmes are still largely at the research stage, but there is nothing to stop you devising your own programme based on similar principles. You should tell your doctor or cardiologist what you are intending to do so you can make sure that you do not overdo it.

Of course, just because symptoms are controlled this does not mean that the underlying problem – i.e. the narrowing and furring of your arteries – has gone away. Even if you do eventually go on to have angioplasty or surgery it is helpful to take a long hard look at your lifestyle to try and prevent atherosclerosis from getting worse and/or to slow its progress. You will find information and advice on how to do this in Chapter 6 which looks at controllable risk factors.

CHAPTER 3

AFTER A HEART ATTACK

'Following your heart attack you should be able to return to a full and active life. For many, life can be better than it was before.'

BHF LEAFLET, LOOKING FORWARD

'Emotionally it was a tremendous shock and afterwards he wasn't prepared for how weak he would feel. He had tremendous psychological barriers. Physically he was better, but emotionally he simply couldn't come to terms with it. Having lost his faith in doctors because he had been told he was all right when he wasn't, he now couldn't believe that he was all right when he was.'

LINDA

HAVING A HEART ATTACK is one of the most frightening events anyone can experience and it will take you time to recover both physically and emotionally. Although the experts generally put the physical recovery time needed at around two to three months there are no hard and fast rules as to how long it takes; everyone is an individual. Take your time and do not feel pressured by what you feel is expected of you either by yourself or other people.

IMMEDIATELY AFTER A HEART ATTACK

In the hours and days following a heart attack you are likely to feel extremely anxious and need a great deal of reassurance. Research shows that six out of ten people who have been admitted to hospital with a suspected heart attack suffer high levels of anxiety. This is especially common in people who were admitted with chest pain of unclear origin which was not diagnosed straight away. Unfortunate though it is, coronary care units are busy places and it is a fact that people occasionally have to wait hours or even days before being given a definite diagnosis and information about their condition. Try to be patient and remember that the main danger has now passed and that you are in the best possible place.

Although you are hungry for information you may feel reluctant to badger busy staff with what you imagine are trivial questions. You may feel obliged to put on a brave face in front of the staff and other patients.

Even if you do ask questions you may find to your dismay that you have forgotten the answers, as Dr Chris Isles, general physician at Dumfries Royal Infirmary points out: 'Patients take in very little when they they have had a heart attack.' Doctors are used to this phenomenon so don't be afraid to ask again if you are at all unclear about anything you have been told or have forgotten something.

One way to get around forgetfulness is to tape record consultations with the doctor. Some hospitals offer you the opportunity to do this anyway. If your hospital is not one of them there is no reason why you should not make your own recording, although of course it is only courteous to explain to the doctor why you are doing it.

DEALING WITH ANXIETY

It is natural to feel anxious after a heart attack but such feelings usually wane rapidly as you take in the fact that you are still alive and begin to feel more confident. High anxiety after a heart attack is partly linked to high levels of the stress hormone adrenalin that are in the body after a heart attack.

It may help to talk over your fears with the staff on the unit. Unfortunately, some medical staff are not always as receptive as they might be, possibly because anxiety is so common, but in this case it helps to know that you have the power to allay your own fears. One way to calm yourself is by relaxation and one very effective method is to listen to a relaxation tape. Studies have shown that listening to such tapes helps lower the heart rate (a sign of anxiety) and also improves long-term recovery. There are numerous commercially available relaxation tapes on the market.

If these measures don't bring your anxiety under control tell the medical staff. A visit from a counsellor or psychotherapist or a brief course of tranquillizers may be what is needed.

TREATMENT OF SIDE EFFECTS

One of the complications of a heart attack which people are often unprepared for is bleeding and bruising arising from the use of 'clotbusters' or thrombolytic drugs used to dissolve the blood clots that are often formed during or immediately after a heart attack. This tendency gradually diminishes as the drugs pass out of the system, but unless you are prepared for it, it can be alarming. You will find more information on drug treatment and side effects in Chapter 4.

GOING HOME AFTER A HEART ATTACK

Much as you have probably been longing to get out of hospital you will probably find your first few weeks at home tiring and bewildering. Many people experience the period after going home from hospital as one of particular stress. This is not surprising. After all, while you were in hospital all your needs were taken care of and you knew that if anything happened a team of doctors and nurses would be immediately at your bedside. Now you have to learn to exist without all this care and back-up. Until you regain your confidence this can be extremely frightening, as Len, who had two heart attacks, points out: 'While I was mollycoddled in hospital I was fine. I was glad to be alive. The nightmare started the day I went home. I was given little information on how to cope on leaving the hospital and what the next few weeks might bring. I felt as if I would never be the same ever again and I became very depressed.'

DEALING WITH EMOTIONAL REACTIONS

The first six weeks after a heart attack are usually a time of conflicting and confusing emotions. Mood swings, tiredness, insomnia, poor concentration and memory, boredom, apathy and anger are all extremely common. Jim remembers: 'I'd started running some time before I had the heart attack. My first reaction was that I'd done all this hard work to get fit and obviously I'd left it too late. I'd always wanted to run, but never got around to it before. Now I'd made the effort and look what had happened. I felt resentful and completely demoralized. I made my wife suffer. I was bad tempered, snapping at the slightest thing. I had great difficulty coming to terms with it and was thoroughly fed up with being in pain (from angina) and not being able to do what I wanted.'

Bear in mind that symptoms such as tiredness may be the result of being out of condition or a side effect of treatment with drugs such as beta-blockers. On the other hand, tiredness can be a feature of depression. You will usually begin to feel more energetic and confident as time goes by. Accepting conflicting emotions and not dwelling on them is the best way to tackle them. It is only if painful emotions impede your recovery or continue for longer than about six weeks that it might be helpful to consult the doctor. You will find more details in Chapter 8.

A GRADUAL PROGRESS

Once you get back home try to give yourself a few days to acclimatize to being back on your own territory. Although your family and friends are naturally eager to see you and hear all about your experience, having too many visitors is tiring. You (or your partner) may need tactfully to dissuade all but your nearest and dearest in the first couple of weeks or so.

Take things slowly and don't attempt to hurl yourself back into your everyday life straight away. It is important to achieve a reasonable balance between rest and activity, building up the amount you do gradually from day to day. This is especially important advice for women whose families sometimes expect them to pick up the reins of running the household from the minute they set foot over the threshold. Encourage other members of your family to share the housework and don't feel guilty if your house is not as spotless as you would want it to be for a while.

EVERY TWINGE IS A HEART ATTACK

Dr Chris Isles, physician at Dumfries Royal Infirmary in Scotland with a special interest in cardiac rehabilitation, observes: 'People who have had a heart attack spend a week in hospital and then they are discharged and told to go home, and they feel every ache and pain.'

Practically all of us experience minor aches and pains from time to time, most of which are insignificant. Usually we are so busy going about our daily lives that we turn a blind eye to them and they disappear. However, when you return home from hospital after a heart attack every minor twinge tends to be magnified.

It is helpful if both you and your nearest and dearest know what is normal. This knowledge will also help you to decide what symptoms you can safely ignore and when it would be a good idea to get medical help. It is exceedingly common, for example, to experience niggling left-sided chest pains, light-headedness and the occasional thump or missed heart beat. Alarming though these are, they are usually quite harmless.

Less common but more serious are severe chest pain, angina on minor exertion, or when you are lying in bed, breathlessness brought on by light exercise and sudden rapid palpitations, especially if you also feel faint. If you experience any of these symptoms contact the doctor or call the cardiac ward.

It is natural to worry about having another heart attack. It is worth bearing in mind that, although the risk of another attack is raised immediately after a heart attack, the risk dwindles as time goes on. By a year after your heart attack you are at no greater risk of having a heart attack than anyone else. Knowing this and being confident that you and your partner could cope in an emergency can help build your confidence.

HOW YOUR FAMILY DOCTOR CAN HELP

Ideally your family doctor will visit you soon after you are discharged from hospital to talk to you about your condition, tell you what the outlook is and advise you about medication. You may have already received advice in hospital but, as has already been observed, it is difficult to take things in if you are worried or in pain.

Your doctor can talk you through again and you should take this opportunity to make sure you understand exactly what is wrong, to acquaint yourself with what drugs you are taking, to find out what medical and ongoing support is available and to air any fears and worries that you have.

The hospital should have been in touch with your family doctor and told him or her that you are home. However it is a good idea to call the surgery yourself and ask the doctor to call if you have not received a visit within a couple of days.

QUESTIONS TO ASK YOUR DOCTOR

Because it is often easy to forget everything you wanted to know the minute you are confronted by anyone in a white coat it is a good idea to make a written list of questions you want to ask. Be tactful about this and don't just thrust it at the doctor and demand that he or she answers your questions, just keep it with you to help jog your memory.

• What is the exact nature of my problem and what caused it?
• What is the condition of my heart and blood vessels now?
• How is my condition likely to progress?
• What drugs are being prescribed? When and how should I take them? How do they act? What should I do if I forget to take them?
• What side effects might I experience? When should I report these to the doctor?
• What can I do to help avoid future problems?
• What symptoms might I expect to experience? Which ones can I safely ignore and which ones should I tell the doctor about?
• How much physical activity can I undertake? How soon can I start to exercise? What sort of exercise, and what pace and level of intensity is safe?
• What sort of support is available in my area for people with heart disease? Is there a local heart support group or chapter, rehabilitation programme and/or specialist cardiac nurse? Are there any local telephone helplines I can call if I need advice?
• Make sure that you remind him or her about any other medication you are being prescribed as well, as drugs may sometimes interact with each other.

Research shows that most of us forget half of what we have been told within five minutes of a consultation with the doctor so it may help to jot down the answers (or tape the consultation as suggested earlier) and ask if there are any leaflets or other written information you can take home.

GETTING TO GRIPS WITH YOUR MEDICATION

Drugs are used for two main reasons after a heart attack: to alleviate symptoms or to prevent a further attack. You may already be familiar with some of the drugs prescribed if you have previously been taking medication for angina and you will find further details in Chapter 4.

You will usually have been given a couple of weeks' supply of medication to tide you over when you get home. You should continue to take this exactly as prescribed, sticking to the same times that you took it in hospital. If in doubt, read the instructions on the packaging or ring the hospital's cardiac helpline.

Once you have returned home the family doctor will usually be in charge of your continuing medication. It is important to make sure you do not run out of medication. When your supplies start to run down, ask for a repeat prescription. You should also tell the doctor about any side effects. Whatever happens never stop taking medication without informing the family doctor or the hospital doctor.

REHABILITATION MATTERS

The weeks and months following your stay in hospital are a time to gradually ease yourself back into everyday life. The technical name for this process is rehabilitation. By the end this period you should be as fit and healthy as possible given any constraints imposed by your condition and feel confident enough to lead a full, active life without being unnecessarily limited by it.

Many hospitals in the UK and most in the US offer a formal rehabilitation programme. This is often based on a four-stage model: stage one – in hospital; stage two – at home; stage three – exercise, relaxation, and advice on managing risk factors such as diet, cholesterol levels and stress; stage four – long-term follow-up and support group.

In practice a more flexible regime tailored to individual needs may be more helpful, as Professor Bob Lewin of the British Heart Foundation's Rehabilitation Research Unit at Hull University argues: 'This sort of model is rather artificial because different people react in different ways at different times. I personally think that people's needs should be assessed. If they need dietary advice they should receive that, if they are not psychologically back to normal after six weeks that should be addressed.' Rehabilitation doesn't have to be a formal process at all. It is something you can do yourself with the support and advice of your medical advisers and your friends and family.

WHY BOTHER WITH REHABILITATION?

There is convincing evidence that taking part in a good rehabilitation programme will help you to get into the exercise habit, increase overall fitness and improve physical and mental health. Even more compellingly, research suggests that people who receive rehabilitation actually have a better chance of surviving a heart attack. Certainly, attending a group helps dispel the idea that after a heart attack you are a permanent invalid, as Howard explains: 'I had expected to be regarded as a patient for the rest of my days. Rehabilitation made me realize I was no longer a patient but an ordinary human being. After I had finished my own rehabilitation I continued to attend as a volunteer. Meeting other people in the same boat and being able to play my part in reassuring them that they were going to be fine was an important part of my own recovery.'

ARE YOU BEING SERVED?

Unfortunately research suggests that in the US fewer than 15 per cent of those who would be eligible actually get to take part in a proper cardiac rehabilitation programme and in the UK the proportion may be even lower.

It also has to be admitted that the content and quality of what is on offer can vary considerably. Ideally a good programme should not just focus on physical training, it should also include advice on how to manage any risk factors in the future and give you emotional support and information on how to relax and think more positively.

One of the biggest problems is that your rehabilitation programme is likely to start several weeks after a heart attack or surgery, leaving you in limbo during the early days and weeks at a time when you are likely to have a strong need for support. 'The time people most need support is just after the event,' says Professor David Thompson of the British Heart Foundation Rehabilitation Research Unit at Hull. 'Unfortunately only a few rehabilitation programmes start on the cardiac ward. Most don't begin until six to eight weeks after the person has returned home, by which time they have started to make adjustments anyway.'

Professor Thompson also argues that the rather blanket approach adopted by some programmes should be abandoned: 'Everyone receives advice on diet even though they may be eating properly, they are told about smoking even if they don't smoke, and given the same programme of exercise even though they would do just as well engaging in regular walking. People should be individually assessed so a programme can be devised to suit their individual needs.'

ASSESSING A REHABILITATION PROGRAMME

If you have been invited to join a rehabilitation programme it is often possible to gauge how likely it is to meet your needs by asking a few leading questions. The following are some ideas:

• **Who organizes the programme?**
A number of different medical staff may be involved. These often include physiotherapists, occupational health nurses, cardiac rehabilitation nurses or cardiac liaison nurses, dietitians and a cardiologist. In many areas health visitors run the programmes and in some places a counsellor, psychologist or even a sex therapist may be invited to give advice about emotional aspects of recovery. In some areas heart support group volunteers may be involved in helping with exercising, making tea and keeping records.

• **Who is eligible for the programme?**
Although cardiac rehabilitation should be offered to everyone with heart disease, you may find that in many centres it is only offered to those who have had a heart attack or heart surgery. You may need to have a word with the cardiac nurse to see if there is a group you can attend. Before enrolling on the programme your condition should have been reviewed and you should have been assessed by the doctor to check whether you are fit to exercise.

• **How many other people will be on the programme?**
The support and camaraderie of others are important features of any rehabilitation programme. Some people remain lifelong friends with others they have met at this time. However, too large

a group may mean that you don't get enough individual attention. Official guidelines generally put the maximum desirable number of attendees at 15.

• **What exercise facilities are there?**
Many programmes are held in a hospital gym. There will usually be a stationary bicycle, a treadmill, and perhaps steps to climb. In the US especially some gyms are splendidly equipped with a vast array of machinery and monitors. Welcome though this is, it isn't strictly necessary and you shouldn't feel deprived if your programme doesn't offer such services. The most vital factors are the knowledge and expertise of the staff involved.

• **How is the programme structured and what does it include?**
Ideally, as we've seen, the programme should be tailored to meet your individual needs. Mike, a support group helper in the UK, explains what happens at his hospital: 'At first the person does a bout of exercise on a walking machine, rowing machine or bike for say two to three minutes and then rests for two to three minutes. If they are not up to that they may just do a minute on a bike at a slow speed and if they aren't up to that they may just walk around the hospital. Each session starts with a warm-up consisting of walking round for two minutes and some gentle stretching. We also include breathing exercises.' Most programmes are graded so that you do progressively more exercise.

• **What provisions are there for handling emergencies?**
One advantage of doing a formal cardiac rehabilitation programme as opposed to simply enrolling in your local gym is that there are trained medical staff present and equipment on hand for dealing with an emergency. If the programme you have enrolled on isn't held in a hospital check that the staff are equipped to deal with emergencies.

• **How will my progress be monitored?**
Any programme worth its salt should include advice on how to measure your progress. By the end of a programme, especially if you have lived a very sedentary life before your heart attack, you'll often be doing what seems like quite strenuous activity. You will usually be taught how to check your own pulse rate to make sure you aren't overdoing it.

• **What other aspects of lifestyle are included?**
Exercise should only be one aspect of rehabilitation. The programme will provice advice on all risk factors: lifestyle, diet, smoking, returning to work and so on.

THE HEART MANUAL – A FRESH APPROACH TO REHABILITATION

Professor Bob Lewin has pioneered a home-based approach to rehabilition based on the psychological technique of cognitive behavioural therapy in which people are encouraged to challenge their false beliefs and practise changing their behaviour.

It involves using a self-help guidebook called *The Heart Manual* together with two cassette tapes which include relaxation exercises and advice for you and your partner. The *Manual* is designed to be prescribed by a doctor or nurse familiar with the person who has had a heart attack and is supervised by someone who has been specially trained in its methods.

The *Manual* is basically a six-week plan for healthy living. It includes lots of information on heart disease designed to combat myths such as the idea that the heart is worn out, plus advice on how to reduce your risk factors, stress management and a graded fitness programme. The programme is interactive so there are lots of charts for you to complete, and refer back to at any time.

Dr Chris Isles, a physician who uses this approach at Dumfries Royal Infirmary, observes: 'People who have had a heart attack fear that their heart muscle is dead and weak. Naturally if you have these words in your head it can paralyse you as far as recovery is concerned. What we try to do is to convert people into "copers". A member of the rehabilitation team goes to visit them in hospital when they have got over the initial attack and follows them through to discharge. When they go home we give them a record card and a follow-up form which tells them which drugs they are on, what risk factors they have and a copy of the *Manual*.'

Although *The Heart Manual* just covers the six weeks after coming home from hospital Dr Isles says that it may take a longer or shorter period than this for people to get back to normal: 'It takes as long as it takes. Some people are not interested; others who are copers to begin with take to it very easily; others need a lot of support.'

DEALING WITH UNMET NEEDS

In a perfect world everyone who has experienced a heart attack would receive high quality aftercare and follow-up. British family doctor Hugh Bethell outlined the ideal scenario in an article in the *British Medical Journal* in 1996: 'Cardiologists in district hospitals could coordinate their aftercare, general practitioners could visit patients soon after discharge; and follow-up in outpatients could be with a doctor of at least registrar status, with encouragment to attend the rehabilitation programme. Finally, general practitioners could organize a follow-up programme that would check on and treat risk factors, review drug treatment and monitor new symptoms.' Unfortunately, as Bethell goes on to point out, too few people who have had a heart attack receive treatment of this quality.

Dr Chris Isles outlines a more typical scenario based on his experience of working on a Coronary Care Unit: 'If they are lucky people get ten minutes with the consultant where there is pressure on them to say everything is fine. Then they go home and again if they are lucky they get ten minutes at the clinic where they have an exercise or treadmill test and then they are expected to get on with it.'

Thanks to the efforts of some healthcare professionals, heart disease charities and pressure groups efforts are now being made in the UK to develop national guidelines and standards for care and rehabilitation. However, there are still gaps in services in many areas.

You may find it especially difficult to get your needs met if you are not the traditional white, middle-aged, male heart patient. A number of studies have shown that women, older people, people of African-Caribbean and Asian origin often miss out. Other people who may benefit from rehabilitation, according to Professor David Thompson, but may not always get it, include people who are especially anxious and cautious as a result of their heart condition, people with medical complications of heart disease, and those who don't live near to a hospital.

If you belong in any of these groups you may need to make an extra effort yourself to ensure that you get the best possible care at this important time in your life. This can be difficult if you are feeling under par or lacking in confidence. In this case your partner or a friend may be able to speak up on your behalf, accompany you when you visit the doctor and find out what services are available in your area. If you don't know anyone who fits the bill you could call a heart charity to see if there is a telephone helpline or cardiac nurse or heart support group in your area who might be able to help.

YOUR FAMILY

In the immediate period surrounding a heart attack or heart surgery you may have been too ill to consider anyone else other than yourself, while in the early stages of recovery you were naturally wrapped up in your own anxieties and fear about your survival. You may have worried about what would happen to your partner and/or children if you died, but beyond that you may not have given much thought to what they were feeling. Once you return home however and start to get back to normal it can help to pay some attention to your family's experiences. Thinking about what they have been through and making an effort to understand some of their emotions will help you to feel closer and enable all concerned to get the support they need.

YOUR PARTNER

'The first night home from hospital was a mixture of happiness that he was back home and terror that if anything went wrong I wouldn't know what to do and there wouldn't be time to call for help. He was equally frightened and neither of us slept much.'

Linda

The first few weeks at home are often extremely stressful for partners. Your partner can be an invaluable ally in your recovery. In fact, Professor David Thompson observes that 'strong partner support is the single most important factor' in buffering the emotional after-effects of a heart attack. However, your partner cannot support you effectively if he or she is overwhelmed by his or her own emotions.

Having a heart attack is a crisis both for the person who had it and for those close to them. Partners often experience a great deal of unacknowledged distress, as Linda observes: 'During this whole period, everyone's attention focused entirely on Len and no one ever asked me how I was feeling or coping. It was a strain and at times quite frightening.'

Like you, your partner may find it hard to come to terms with what has happened. He or she may experience a similar mixture of emotions. These can include grief, depression, anxiety, anger and a feeling that life has spiralled frighteningly out of control. Because you are the one who experienced the actual attack he or she may feel unable to share these emotions for fear of upsetting or worrying you. 'Although I tried to be supportive and cheerful,' Linda says, 'it was an extremely exhausting and demanding period. We would have dearly liked to have someone to turn to for comfort and support who had either experienced it themselves or at least understood and had the time to talk to either of us.'

SUPPORT GROUPS AND HELPLINES

Feeling able to talk over the experience and confronting fears is important for your partner. However your partner may feel that you have enough on your plate without burdening you with his or her concerns. Having someone in whom they can confide such as a good friend or relative is invaluable at this time. Nevertheless, friends and relatives, however supportive, do not always have accurate facts about heart disease. For this reason it often helps for partners to be able to talk with medical advisers, a cardiac nurse or support group helper.

'In many cases people's fears are a result of ignorance. Once they are aware of the facts they are able to relax and feel more confident,' explains British Heart Foundation nurse Karen Caffrey.

Some hospitals have a special Cardiac Helpline which former patients and their partners can call if they have any anxieties, and some have British Heart Foundation nurses who visit you at home and help you and your partner deal with any worries and concerns. If you or your partner need more concentrated support or counselling this can be organized too.

However much help and support you get from those around you no one understands what it is like to have a heart attack as well as someone else who has experienced one. Once the initial recovery period is over you may find it helpful to join a support group. You will find details of these in Chapter 8.

CHAPTER 4

MEDICAL TREATMENTS FOR HEART DISEASE

'The introduction of a whole range of different drugs in the past few years which improve blood flow, lessen the extent of damage in a heart attack and lower cholesterol levels has played a significant part in reducing the need for surgery and improving the quality of life for people with heart disease.'

BELINDA LINDEN, NURSE ADVISER, BRITISH HEART FOUNDATION

MANY PEOPLE WITH DISEASED ARTERIES have their condition controlled by drugs alone. Others may eventually need surgery. This chapter is intended to give you some idea of how the drugs you may have been prescribed work and some of the side effects that you may experience.

TYPES OF DRUGS

Drugs used for heart disease fall into two broad types: those used for primary prevention, in other words drugs used to prevent coronary artery disease and correct specific risk factors such as high cholesterol, and those used for secondary prevention, to treat existing symptoms of heart disease such as angina. Over the past few years a number of very effective drugs aimed at secondary prevention have made an appearance. These are making a real difference in helping people with heart disease to stay healthier for longer and can sometimes actually reverse some of the symptoms of disease.

Within these broad types there are numerous different drugs, which may seem confusing, but most of them fall into a few well-defined categories. Although the drugs in each category work in broadly similar ways there are often subtle differences in action between them.

How well a particular drug works depends on several factors including your age, sex, weight and any other health problems you might have. Your doctor will take these into account in trying to prescribe a medication which is most suited to your needs.

DEALING WITH SIDE EFFECTS

All drugs involve costs as well as benefits and those used for heart disease are no exception. It is as well to know what these are, so that if you develop any unexpected effects you can report them to the doctor.

When thinking about side effects it is vital to bear in mind that any substance which is chemically active (and this includes preparations you can buy over the counter and 'natural' remedies such as herbal treatments) have side effects. In the case of any particular drug the doctor will try to weigh the benefits for your heart against the disadvantages of any potentially harmful effects. 'All drugs can have minor side effects,' says Belinda Linden, nurse adviser to the BHF. 'It does not necessarily mean that they are harmful or should not be taken. This may only be advisable when side effects are severe or if the doctor feels that the risks of the side effects outweigh the benefit of the drug.' If you find you are not being helped by the drugs, never just stop taking them as sudden withdrawal can make angina worse. Tell the doctor so he or she can taper your dose off gradually.

It can be alarming to read long lists of side effects, but it is worth bearing in mind that they don't affect everybody and that many subside once your body has become acclimatized to the drug. Some side effects are a nuisance rather than serious and can be treated by simple self-help methods. Constipation, for example, is a side effect of many heart drugs, but can often be solved simply by eating more fruit and vegetables and drinking more fluids.

If you have been prescribed a particular drug which doesn't suit you and is causing you unacceptable side effects, don't just grin and bear it – go back and ask the doctor if he or she can prescribe something else. Individuals react differently to different drugs and it can sometimes take time before the particular drug or combination of drugs which is best for you is found.

MEDICATION CHECKLIST

- Make sure you understand what each drug prescribed is for and what side effects are normal
- Make sure you know how many times a day you need to take the drug and how it should be taken e.g. dissolved under the tongue, taken with water, sprayed and so on. If you are taking several different types of tablets it is possible to get special dispensers which make life easier
- Always take medication exactly as it is prescribed. Do not take other people's medicines
- Check the packet for any special instructions and make sure you don't keep any tablets beyond their use-by date. Nitroglycerin tablets, for example, lose their strength quickly once the bottle has been opened and need to be replaced after six to eight weeks
- If in any doubt about any medication you have been prescribed check with the doctor or pharmacist

Not everyone is interested in knowing a great deal of detail about the drugs they have been prescribed. Nevertheless you may find it helpful to have some idea of the purpose of whichever medication you are taking and how your body may react. The chart on page 171 (Appendix 2) lists the drugs most commonly prescribed for various heart conditions.

BETA-BLOCKERS

Beta-blockers, medically known as **beta-adrenoceptor blocking drugs,** work by blocking the action of stress hormones such as adrenalin that make your heart beat faster. They slow the heart rate, lower blood pressure and reduce the work the heart has to do. This in turn reduces the amount of oxygen the heart needs to do its job and so improves its ability to deal with exertion.

Beta-blockers are used to treat high blood pressure and to prevent angina, although they work too slowly to be used to give instant relief in an angina attack. Some kinds of beta-blockers are effective in reducing the chance of having another heart attack in people who have had an uncomplicated heart attack, but they are not usually prescribed if the heart muscle is very damaged as they may weaken its pumpimg ability even further.

There are many different types of beta-blocker and no one formulation is preferable, but some people respond better to one than another. If you don't get on with one that has been prescribed, don't be afraid to tell the doctor, who may be able to prescribe a different formulation.

Side effects

Carefully used, beta-blockers are usually quite safe. Because they don't just block adrenalin receptors in the heart, however, they can sometimes trigger side effects in other organs or tissues. The most common minor side effects are feeling more tired than usual and cold hands and feet caused by the drugs constricting blood vessels to the extremities. Some people experience sleep disturbances and nightmares.

More seriously, beta-blockers can spark off asthma because they constrict the small airways in the lungs, so they aren't suitable if you have asthma or any other illness affecting the airways. They are also not recommended if you have narrowed arteries in your legs and intermittent claudication, as they can make this worse.

Beta-blockers are also unsuitable for people with diabetes who are prone to **hypoglycaemia** (low blood sugar) because they can mask the problem. If your diabetes is well controlled there should be no problem, though the doctor may prescribe what are known as 'selective' beta-blockers. The doctor will also be very careful if you have heart failure and will only prescribe beta-blockers if your condition is under control.

Other less frequent side effects can include nausea, diarrhoea, dry eyes, skin rashes, pins and needles in the fingers, and sexual problems such as inability to get an erection. Changing to a different type of beta-blocker may solve these problems.

CALCIUM-CHANNEL BLOCKERS

Calcium-channel blockers, or **calcium antagonists**, as they are also called, reduce the amount of calcium ions entering the muscle cells of the heart and arteries, causing them to relax. This in turn opens up the arteries, boosting the blood supply to the heart and reducing the work the heart has to do in pumping the blood around your body. Many only have to be taken once a day and they are often used in combination with other drugs such as beta-blockers.

Different calcium-channel blockers have different modes of action. Some, such as verapamil, used for the treatment of angina, high blood pressure and irregular heart rhythm, slow the heart rate, so should not be used with beta-blockers. Others, such as nifedipine, also used for angina and high blood pressure, may speed up the heart rate. The doctor will take all aspects of your medical condition into account before choosing the most suitable one for you.

Side effects
Because they open up the arteries all calcium-channel blockers may cause flushing, dizziness, faintness and headache, though these usually become less troublesome after a few days. Ankle swelling is another common side effect. You may experience constipation if you are taking verapamil. Some calcium-channel blockers may cause stomach upsets of various kinds and very occasionally rashes and depression. As with other drugs, research continues to improve safety and reduce side effects of calcium-channel blockers and your doctor will want to weigh up all the pros and cons before prescribing them.

NITRATES

Nitrates work by relaxing the muscles in the walls of the blood vessels, so reducing the work that the left ventricle of the heart has to do. Nitrates are also useful in preventing long-term angina, although they tend to become less effective over time.

A tablet of **glyceryl trinitrate (GTN)** placed under the tongue or a couple of bursts from an aerosol spray is one of the most effective ways of combatting an attack of angina quickly, although effects only lasts for around 20 to 30 minutes. If you have stable (predictable) angina the doctor will usually tell you to take a tablet before any exertion that normally brings on an attack.

Nitrates also come in other forms. **Buccal** tablets, placed between the upper lip and the gum, are slow-release preparations which work over four to six hours. Another alternative is a **nitroglycerin patch**, which you stick on your chest. The body absorbs the drug through the skin and the patch can be worn all day long. Unfortunately, some people quickly build up a tolerance to patches and their effectiveness is lowered. If the doctor suspects you have developed a tolerance he or she will usually suggest that you remove the patch for several hours each day.

Side effects
Unwanted side effects include flushing, a throbbing headache, dizziness and faintness. Although all the different preparations can cause them, these side effects tend to be most common with tablets. For this reason it's a good idea to sit down when you first take a tablet in case you feel faint. The good news is that such effects usually wane with continued use.

THROMBOLYTIC DRUGS – 'CLOTBUSTERS'

The use of clotbusters or thrombolytics has dramatically reduced the risk of dying of a heart attack in the past decade. Given after a heart attack starts they act to break up clots, restore blood flow through the blocked artery and reduce damage to the heart muscle.

Clotbusters must be administered as soon as possible after a heart attack begins because, as we've seen, the longer the heart muscle is deprived of its blood supply the more damage is done. Prompt use of a clotbuster can change a potentially severe heart attack into a mild one and can sometimes avert any damage whatsoever.

The clotbuster most often used is called **streptokinase**. It is given intravenously for an hour and after that you'll be given aspirin.

Side effects
As clotbusters dissolve clots, one of their more serious potential side effects is that they can cause serious bleeding. That means if you have recently had an operation or suffered bleeding from another cause you won't be prescribed them. Part of the skill of the doctor in the coronary unit is to weigh up the risks carefully against the benefits.

ASPIRIN

In the past few years this everyday painkiller has been found to have a real role in reducing the risk of dying in a heart attack. Taking an aspirin a day after a heart attack helps prevent death in the immediate aftermath and after that continuing treatment is extremely effective in preventing a recurrence. Low-dose aspirin is now prescribed for all patients with coronary heart disease unless there is any special reason not to do so.

Aspirin works by reducing the stickiness of the blood and so combatting clotting. It can also be used if you have angina, and helps prevent narrowing in the vein grafts used in bypass operations.

Side effects

One of the beauties of aspirin is that it has so few side effects. However, it should be used with caution if you are asthmatic, as it can provoke an attack of wheezing, and should be avoided if you have a peptic ulcer, suffer from haemophilia or other bleeding disorder. Asprin sometimes causes indigestion, nausea, vomiting and constipation. Such problems can usually be overcome by using a lower dose or a coated preparation to help avoid irritating the lining of the stomach.

ANTI-COAGULANTS

Anti-coagulant drugs are designed to thin the blood and prevent it from clotting. They are given intravenously to prevent clotting straight away and also prescribed as tablets to prevent long-term clotting.

Warfarin is usually used for people with diseases of the heart valves or who have had an artificial valve inserted, and for people who have atrial fibrillation.

Anti-coagulants are also used for treating deep vein thrombosis (clots in the leg veins) to prevent these from travelling to the lungs where they can cause a potentially fatal pulmonary embolism.

If you are prescribed an anti-clotting drug you will need to have regular blood tests to make sure that the clotting activity of the blood is kept within safe limits. It is also important to tell the doctor or pharmacist before you take any other medications, either prescribed or over-the-counter. This is because anti-coagulants can interact with other drugs such as antibiotics, aspirin, cimedtidine (used to treat ulcers) and drugs used to treat arthritis, gout, epilepsy, raised cholesterol levels and disorders of heart rhythm.

Side effects
The drugs need to be very finely balanced according to a measurement known as the **International Normalized Ratio** or **INR**. It is very important to get the dosage exactly right, and this can sometimes take a little time, as Carolyn found: 'I came out of hospital with clear instructions only to let the INR reach a certain level. The doctors and nurses from my local surgery took blood samples to determine if the warfarin should be upped or lowered but they didn't get the level the same as I had been told it should be in hospital. They say most people should keep at around 2.5 to 3 but mine had to be 4.5. When I mentioned it they said it didn't matter, but I didn't feel happy so I phoned the hospital and spoke to the surgeon. He said you must make them realize it has got to be this level. It was difficult but I persevered.'

If you are prescribed an anti-coagulant you should always carry an Anti-coagulant Card so that if you need medical attention the staff will know that you are taking anti-coagulants.

ACE INHIBITORS

ACE inhibitors – or **angiotensin-converting enzyme inhibitors** to give them their full name – work by blocking the effects of a hormone called angiotension which causes the blood vessels to constrict. By opening up the blood vessels ACE inhibitors improve blood flow and decrease the amount of work the heart has to do. They are most effective when combined with diuretics to reduce congestion in the lungs.

ACE inhibitors are used to treat and prevent heart failure and to lower blood pressure. They are particularly useful for treating high blood pressure in people with diabetes, although for reasons not fully understood they have been found to be less effective in African-Caribbean people.

Side effects
The main problem with ACE inhibitors is that in some people they can cause a dramatic drop in blood pressure when they are first prescribed. For this reason the doctor will probably suggest that you take the first dose in bed, so you will not fall over if your blood pressure does fall.

You should be started on a low dose which is increased gradually. If the doctor anticipates a particular risk or problems, it may be suggested that you are admitted to hospital so you can be treated promptly if your blood pressure drops too low.

ACE inhibitors are not recommended for people with kidney disease as in some cases they can affect the kidneys further. All patients who are taking ACE inhibitors will have periodic blood tests to check their kidney function and prevent problems occurring.

Some ACE inhibitors may cause changes in taste, a dry, hacking cough, skin rashes and occasionally may spark a severe allergic reaction. If you experience the latter you should contact your doctor or go to the hospital without delay.

ANTI-ARRHYTHMIC DRUGS

These are drugs designed to correct irregularities in heart rhythms. Although beta-blockers and the calcium antagonist verapamil may be useful in this context there are several others which are used almost solely for correcting arrhythmias. It is especially important to take the drugs exactly as prescribed because the effectiveness of this group of drugs depends on maintaining a precise amount in your blood stream.

Digoxin, a synthetic drug derived from the foxglove (digitalis), is used for treating the arrhythmia known as atrial fibrillation (see page 29). The condition may accompany heart failure. Digoxin slows and strengthens the heartbeat, which may be sufficient to relieve breathlessness and palpitations, but it does not always restore a regular beat and other drugs or treatments may be needed to normalize the heart beat.

Side effects
Although they are generally well tolerated, all the anti-arrhythmic drugs used can cause side effects so it is especially important to report any unusual symptoms to your doctor. Your doctor may want to admit you to hospital when the drugs are first introduced so the effects on your heart can be monitored.

Amiodarone is very effective at controlling some abnormal heart rhythms, but can be liable to produce side effects. As well as some of the more familiar ones such as headaches, flushing and dizziness it can – rarely – cause inflammation of the liver and lungs. It may also affect the functioning of the thyroid gland which controls the metabolism and so affect all the body's systems. Taking amiodarone can also make you more prone to sunburn and result in a slate-blue skin tone, so it is especially important to use a high SPF sun barrier and wear a hat when going out in the sun.

Anti-arrhythmic drugs can sometimes react with other drugs so it is especially important to make sure all your doctors know exactly which drugs you are taking if you are prescribed any new medication for any reason whatsoever.

Digoxin can cause appetite loss and nausea and, less often, vomiting, painful or (occasionally) enlarged breasts, rash, palpitation and fainting.

LIPID-LOWERING DRUGS/ANTI-CHOLESTEROL DRUGS

Lipid-lowering drugs work either by raising levels of 'good' HDL cholesterol, lowering triglyceride levels and/or lowering levels of 'bad' LDL cholesterol. The most recent research suggests that they can dramatically slow the progression of narrowing of the arteries and may sometimes even cause the build-up of plaque to be reversed in people with high cholesterol levels.

The introduction of the latest family of cholesterol-lowering drugs, known as **statins**, has led to a rash of new studies. At present the jury is still out on whether cholesterol-lowering drugs should be used in people with high cholesterol levels but no symptoms of heart disease, but there is now overwhelming evidence that people who have existing heart disease and high cholesterol levels despite a strict diet low in saturated fats, do benefit from cholesterol-lowering drugs.

The European Society of Cardiology now recommends treatment with cholesterol-lowering drugs if cholesterol levels remain high after three to six months of changed diet. If you are prescribed these drugs you should not abandon your attempts to lower your cholesterol level by a low-fat diet, exercise and giving up smoking, however, as continuing to eat a high-fat diet can counteract their beneficial effects. Appendix 2 includes a chart of lipid-lowering drugs, with details of how they are taken and their common side effects.

CHAPTER 5

DEALING WITH SURGERY AND OTHER PROCEDURES

'The stairs seemed like Mount Everest, the hallway two miles long and on those first walks outside in the cold winter's air the street seemed endless. So was this life after bypass? I felt as if I would never be the same ever again and I became very depressed.'

LEN

'I used to suffer badly with intermittent claudication in my legs when I walked. Since my bypass, unless I really go over the top, I never suffer from it. I feel I've been given my life back.'

JOHN

IF ANGINA CANNOT BE TREATED BY DRUGS or if your arteries are badly blocked you may be offered further help in the form of a procedure such as balloon angioplasty or heart surgery. This chapter gives a rundown of the most common procedures involved and how to cope both before and afterwards.

In the past people with heart disease were usually treated first with drugs and then if the condition progressed with bypass surgery. Today a whole range of new procedures designed to widen the arteries and clear away atheroma have widened the choice tremendously. These techniques are known as **interventional cardiology**. They have the huge advantage of being able to be carried out under local anaesthetic, making recovery time speedier and less painful than after surgery. And, of course, because they do not involve the chest being opened up there is also no scar.

INTERVENTIONAL PROCEDURES

BALLOON ANGIOPLASTY

The most common and well-known procedure is balloon angioplasty, or, as doctors call it, **percutaneous transluminal coronary angioplasty (PTCA)**. A long fine catheter with a tiny, deflated, sausage-shaped balloon at its tip is passed into an artery through a small sheath in the groin (the skin is numbed first with a local anaesthetic). This is pushed through under X-ray vision until the narrowed part of the coronary artery is reached. The balloon is then inflated at high pressure, compressing the fatty deposits of atherosclerotic plaque against the artery walls. This widens the artery so more blood can flow through. The balloon is then deflated and withdrawn. The doctor then does a repeat angiogram to see how successful the procedure has been and the catheter is then pulled out as well.

Balloon angioplasty is extremely successful, with most patients experiencing relief from angina. It may be the treatment for you if your heart function is basically good but you have blockages in one or two arteries and angina that is not being controlled by drugs. It is also sometimes used for people with silent ischaemia who have had a heart attack and been found to have one or two narrowed arteries. Carolyn remembers: 'The only thing I felt was a slight tickling in the groin and a slight tugging. There was no pain – I didn't feel the catheter going through the artery – but I felt a slight tightening in my throat when they inflated the balloon, a bit like indigestion but not severe. Afterwards there was discomfort in the groin area and it was quite bruised.'

OTHER INTERVENTIONAL TECHNIQUES

You may also be offered one of a variety of other techniques. The most common is the insertion of one or more **stents**, tiny 'scaffolds' of wire mesh placed into the artery to hold it open. Other more high-tech options include **laser angioplasty**, which uses a laser instead of or as well as a balloon to melt through the fatty deposits and plaque. In a procedure called an **atherectomy** a high-speed cutting drill shaves plaque off the artery wall. However, balloon angioplasty remains the most common treatment of choice.

IN HOSPITAL

Immediately after having a procedure such as angioplasty or having a stent inserted you will be told to stay in bed and keep your leg as straight as possible to limit the risk of bleeding. The medical staff will keep a careful eye on you during the first few hours after the operation. The sheath through which the catheter was introduced into the artery in your groin is removed, usually on the same day. A small dressing will be placed over the wound and you will be asked to stay in bed for another few hours. After this rest you will usually be able to go home.

DEALING WITH A STENT

After having a stent inserted you will need to take an anti-platelet drug. Platelets are red blood cells which play a role in forming blood clots which, without treatment, can be inclined to form on stents. Patients are usually given aspirin and ticlopidine, another anti-platelet drug that works in a slightly different way from aspirin. The ticlopidine is given for about a month but the aspirin continues indefinitely. Several new types of anti-platelet drugs are being researched.

AT HOME

Physically, recovery is much speedier after having a procedure such as angioplasty or a stent than it is after a bypass, which, after all, is major surgery. You can expect to feel a bit sore and have some bruising around the leg wound. The area may feel quite hard to the touch at first but should return to normal within a couple of weeks. If the wound becomes more painful or if bruising worsens or the wound starts to bleed or ooze see your doctor. Otherwise simple painkillers should combat any pain.

You may also experience some discomfort and bruising in the chest. Again this can be helped by taking a painkiller. Some people experience angina after angioplasty in which case you should use any drugs you have previously been prescribed. However, if you are getting angina regularly you should contact the doctor. Similarly, if you experience chest pain that is not associated with exertion and/or suspect you may be having a heart attack you should also call the doctor or call the emergency services (see Appendix 1).

Emotionally, even though you have not had a major operation, it can still can take some time to come to terms with what you have been through, especially if the procedure was carried out as an emergency or soon after a diagnosis of heart disease. Carolyn says: 'After I came out of hospital having had the stent put in my confidence went out of the window and it's taken a long time to get back to normal.' You will find more details about dealing with emotions in Chapter 8.

EVERYDAY LIFE

How soon you can start taking up the threads of your everyday life again will depend on whether the procedure you had done was a straightforward, planned operation or whether you went into hospital as an emergency. Usually, if your procedure was planned, you will be able to start driving around a week afterwards, provided you are feeling well.

Other activities will depend very much on your individual case. You should usually be able to take up any sports you play again within about four weeks, though you should discuss this with the doctor before you leave hospital. You can start having sex again as soon as you feel ready (see Chapter 8). You can go on holiday or fly too as soon as you like (unless you have had a recent heart attack) but it would be best to discuss this with your doctor. Some people are advised to wait until after their six-week check-up with the consultant. You should discuss with the doctor when it would be advisable to return to work, too.

HEART SURGERY

The main operation used to treat coronary artery disease is the **coronary artery bypass graft**, shortened to **CABG** by doctors, but usually known to the rest of us as a **heart bypass**. In the UK over 21,000 people have heart bypasses each year; in the US 318,000 people are operated upon.

A heart bypass is just what is sounds like: a way literally of bypassing a blocked coronary artery in the heart. The operation involves taking another blood vessel from somewhere else in your body such as a leg vein, a vein from the arm or, more usually today, the internal mammary artery that runs inside the chest wall, and 'grafting' this on to the blocked coronary artery. The number of grafts you need will depend on how many of the diseased arteries are blocked. Although you may only need one graft most people need two, three or even four. In these cases the terms double, triple or quadruple bypass are used.

The second most common type of heart operation is **valve surgery**, accounting for 5000 in the UK and in the US some 60,000 heart operations each year. It is used to repair or replace valves that have become narrowed or leaky.

Occasionally, the surgeon can repair the valve without replacing it. However usually the diseased valve will be cut out and another inserted in its place. The new valve may be a pig valve or a homograft, a human valve, or be made from an artificial material such as metal or plastic. In this case you will have to take anti-coagulant medication to prevent blood clots from developing on the valve's surfaces.

Valvuloplasty, a technique similar to angioplasty in which a balloon is inserted to widen a narrowed heart valve, is occasionally used.

The third type of heart surgery you may undergo is **heart transplantation**. Despite all the publicity in the media about heart transplants, it is in fact a much less common operation than the other two. It involves removing your own diseased heart and replacing it with a healthy one from a donor. In the past transplant operations sometimes failed because the patient's body rejected the transplanted heart. Today, thanks to new drugs which prevent this happening, heart transplants are very successful, although the shortage of donor organs limits its wider use.

HOW YOU MIGHT FEEL

If you have been told you need heart surgery you may experience a number of conflicting emotions: shock, fear, misery, relief that at last something is being done, especially if angina or breathlessness is interfering badly with your everyday life, or simple disbelief.

Howard says: 'I'd started having angina much more frequently; just walking to my room I had to slow down. I saw the consultant who put me on a treadmill. When he came back to the room, he said "Wrap yourself in cotton wool and I'll see you in a week's time for an angiogram." My wife accompanied me. When I'd had the test the consultant said, "It's very serious; you must come straight into hospital." My wife thinks it's a good thing it happened so quickly. I was very worried but I was reassured after the initial shock.'

Sometimes people feel sure that the doctor has got it wrong. This 'denial' is often the mind's way of coming to terms with difficult information. It usually passes as you realize that an operation is necessary.

If you continue to find it hard to accept that an operation is needed it may help to talk to your doctor and get him or her to explain exactly why it is thought to be necessary and what the benefits are likely to be. Len's wife, Linda, recalls: 'When Len was told he needed a virtually immediate operation he said, "It's not that urgent, is it?" The doctor said, "No, you could live another year or you could have an argument with a traffic warden when you walk out of here and it would be enough to trigger a heart attack." '

RELIEVING ANXIETY

Research shows that anxiety is usually highest before surgery but drops rapidly after the operation. Knowing what to expect helps a lot. You should be invited to the hospital to meet the surgeon who should explain the results of any tests you have had, explain what is involved in the surgery, what benefits you can expect to gain and give you some idea of how successful surgery is expected to be. Your partner may like to attend this meeting too, so if he or she is not invited it may be worth asking if they can attend.

As suggested earlier, it may help to tape record this meeting. Alternatively many hospitals provide written information about what to expect and the various heart charities also produce useful information leaflets.

Some people, of course, prefer to know as little as possible and leave it all up to the medical staff. There is no need to feel guilty about feeling like this. However, if you are at all unsure about anything it is a good idea to discuss it with your doctor or contact the cardiac team at the hospital where you are to have your operation.

Bear in mind that heart surgeons carry out such operations every day and that today they are virtually always extremely successful and safe. Most people who have had heart surgery say they are very pleased to have had their operation and many say they feel they have been given a new lease of life – studies show that seven out of ten people would have the operation again!

WAITING FOR TREATMENT

In some areas long waiting lists mean that it may well be some time before you can have your operation. During this time try to live as normally as possible. You may find the advice on dealing with angina given in Chapter 2 useful. Nevertheless, the time spent waiting can be somewhat stressful and you may experience mood swings and feel angry, irritated and frightened.

Jim believes that it pays to be persistent: 'Waiting was very frustrating. I'm someone who likes to be in charge of my life, it probably comes from being in industry. I rang the consultant's secretary a couple of times and found her very sympathetic. Some people tend to shrink from doing that, but I found it helped me to feel in control. If you sit back and wait, you'll wait forever.'

Sometimes, though, no matter how persistent you are, you simply have to wait until your name reaches the top of the waiting list. It can help you feel more in control if you use this time to look at your lifestyle and start tackling risk factors like stopping smoking, cutting down on fatty foods and losing weight if you need to. Getting as fit as you can before your operation will help your body to deal with it better and will also help ensure your recovery is as speedy as possible.

MAKING PRACTICAL ARRANGEMENTS

In most areas you will be notified when you have to go into hospital a week or two beforehand. You may be told to stop certain drugs beforehand – check with your doctor or consultant.

During the run-up to your operation you will also need to make practical arrangements: someone to look after you when you go home, arranging for someone to keep an eye on your house if it is to be empty, getting someone to look after any pets you have and packing your bag. You will usually be given a list of what you need to take in by the hospital. Don't forget to have some small change for telephone calls. It may also be a good idea to pack a relaxation tape and a tape recorder. The following advice is based on information contained in London's St George's Healthcare Trust leaflet, *Preparing for Heart Surgery*:

- Discuss who will be taking you home from hospital.
- If you are being driven home by a member of the family or a friend it is helpful to get a small cushion to place between your chest and seat belt, as by law you still have to wear a seat belt after your operation.
- In the first two weeks after you get home it is helpful to have a family member with you to give general support. They may need to arrange to take time off work.
- Some people like to go to a convalescence home after their operation. Such homes are almost always private. Staff at the hospital may be able to advise you on one in your area.

IN HOSPITAL

You will usually be admitted the day before your operation and will usually have to have a chest X-ray, ECGs, blood and urine tests to make sure that the doctor has a full picture of your current health. You will also be asked about your drinking and smoking habits and any drugs you are taking regularly. It is important to be completely honest as they may affect your recovery.

The anaesthetist will usually visit you some time during the day or evening before your operation to explain what is involved, your chest will be washed with an antiseptic solution and – if you are a man and have a hairy chest – will be shaved. You will not be able to have anything to eat after midnight because anaesthesia is safer on an empty stomach.

On the morning of your operation you will be given a mild tranquillizer to help you keep calm, electrodes will be attached to you so your heart can be monitored throughout the operation. You will be given a general anaesthetic (the last thing you will remember is likely to be the anaesthetic drug given in your veins). Intravenous lines will be inserted into the veins of your arm or wrist to allow the anaesthetist to drip drugs directly into your bloodstream and to keep your body fluid level balanced. One of these lines is threaded all the way up to the vena cava, a large vein near the heart. Another allows the staff to monitor your blood pressure and oxygen level in your arteries. You will also have catheters (fine tubes) inserted into your neck vein to monitor blood flow and arterial pressure and also a urinary catheter to collect urine (a sign of how well the kidneys are functioning). A tube called an endotracheal tube is inserted into your windpipe. This is connected to a respirator, a machine that breathes for you. Another tube called a nasogastric tube is inserted to collect stomach fluids to avoid your being sick.

AFTER THE OPERATION

You will spend the first few days after surgery in the ICU, the **intensive care unit**, where sophisticated equipment and monitors will be used to keep a check on your well-being. Your family will be able to visit you there, although you are likely to be sleepy from the anaesthetic. You will not be able to speak either because of the endotracheal tube. You will usually be taken off the respirator within a few hours of surgery and all the intravenous drips and catheters will usually be removed over the next day or two.

You can usually expect to spend around seven days in hospital although the exact length of time will depend on how well your recovery period goes. In some hospitals in both the UK and the US surgeons are using a special 'fast-track' recovery programme designed to cut down the need for a stay in intensive care and the number of days spent in hospital after a bypass. As a rough rule of thumb people who have had bypasses tend to recover quicker than those who have had valve surgery. Your age comes into it too: older people tend to need longer to recover than younger ones, although this is by no means always the case.

Afterwards you may remember little about the operation and the first few days afterwards. As Howard recalls: 'I was conscious of being in intensive care and I remember I found visitors very tiring. I was pleased because my wife used to rescue me. I felt very tired and slept every afternoon and I had to sit down to shave. I was disinterested in food and I was told I was very miserable until the day I came home.'

SOME PRACTICALITIES

You will usually have been taught some simple breathing exercises by the physiotherapist before the operation to help clear phlegm that may have accumulated in your lungs as a result of the anaesthetic and told to cough to clear the phlegm. This may be uncomfortable, so support your chest wound by placing your hands on either side of your rib cage or by placing one hand over the other in the centre of your chest when you cough. You may also have been taught shoulder exercises to relieve stiffness and aching in your chest and shoulders and leg exercises to keep your circulation moving in your legs and help avoid a blood clot from forming.

DEALING WITH THE CHEST WOUND

During heart surgery your breast bone or sternum is cut to allow the surgeon access to your heart. The stitches inserted afterwards are soluble and will dissolve after two or three weeks as the wound heals. Once initial healing has taken place, after a couple of days or so, the dressing will usually be removed as exposure to air encourages better healing. If the incision continues to ooze it may be covered with a dressing until it is dry.

You should avoid pressure on the scar and will probably find it more comfortable to wear loose clothes for several weeks and maybe longer. Women may experience chafing from wearing a bra. In this case either leave your bra off for a while or invest in a soft, unwired one.

DEALING WITH PAIN AND DISCOMFORT

As after any operation you can expect to feel some pain. In the early days after your operation you will be given painkillers. Do not be afraid to tell the staff if you are in pain and if you do not find the drugs you have been given effective don't just grin and bear it. Pain relief is more effective if pain is quelled early on rather than allowing it to take hold. Sylvia recalls: 'There were times when the pain was dreadful but each day is an improvement and as you get better you feel better in body and mind.'

'Post-operatively my sternum was terribly sore,' says Gill. 'I couldn't wear a bra and it's only now, a year later, that I've started wearing one again. My legs were painful too and that was rather a shock. Even now they swell up and I can't stand still for long.'

Pain is always worse if you are afraid, so knowing what pain to expect and what you can do to relieve it should ensure that you do not suffer unduly. It usually takes around three months for complete healing to take place after heart surgery.

You may experience pain in the chest or the leg or arm where the blood vessel has been removed. Your leg may also swell slightly. Wearing an elastic support stocking and keeping your feet up when you sit down for the first few weeks after your operation will help. Howard observes: 'It took a good three months before I could do what I wanted to do. The wound from the leg held me back because of the pain. I used to put my leg up and keep it up.' You may experience numbness and pins and needles around the scar. It is nothing to worry about and usually goes away of its own accord. You can aid the healing process and avoid discomfort by making sure that you don't overdo it especially in the first six weeks after your operation.

In the first few weeks you can expect to experience muscle pain especially in the centre of your chest, neck, back and arms where the ligaments and muscles have been stretched during the operation. This is normal and will gradually fade as the scar heals.

You may find you feel especially stiff and uncomfortable first thing in the morning in which case it can help to do the exercises you have been taught.

If what you are suffering is discomfort rather than actual pain, doing something distracting such as reading a book, calling a friend or going for a walk may help. If pain is so severe you cannot ignore it you should tell the doctor, as there are various painkilling drugs that can be prescribed to help. There are also techniques of pain management, including relaxation techniques, that will help you feel more in control of any pain you may be experiencing. These days, with effective techniques of pain relief, there is no need for anyone to put up with severe pain either while they are in hospital or at home.

GOING HOME

Much of what has been said in Chapter 3 about recovering from a heart attack applies to people who have undergone surgery. Mild depression and anxiety are normal and feelings tend to fluctuate from day to day depending on how you are feeling physically.

It is natural to feel more positive some days than others, especially in the immediate aftermath of an operation. However, slowly but surely you should feel better and stronger. One way to get around ups and downs of emotions, as suggested by the British Heart Foundation, is to take a longer view of your progress and view it from week to week rather than from day to day. Gill emphasizes the importance of allowing yourself plenty of time. 'They tell you it's going to be all right in six weeks, but it isn't. In my experience you don't feel back to normal for a long time. My sternum took 18 months to stop hurting. Now everything's fine. The scars have healed brilliantly, they hardly show at all. I had to be careful with sunbathing for the first couple of summers because if you expose the scar tissue to the sun it doesn't heal properly. That was something one of the nurses told me, so I used a sun lotion factor 20 or total block. Now it's OK.'

HOW SUCCESSFUL IS BYPASS SURGERY?

According to the British Heart Foundation between 80 and 85 per cent of people who have a bypass experience immediate and lasting pain relief. In most of the remaining 15 to 20 per cent the pain is much improved.

It has to be said that some people who undergo bypass surgery do not experience complete pain relief, although often they do feel a significant benefit. The surgeon will usually advise you beforehand if this is likely to be your experience.

Furthermore, as a bypass does nothing to correct the underlying cause of your heart disease, i.e. the furring and narrowing of your arteries, pain may come back as the disease progresses. It is estimated that this happens in approximately 5 per cent of people every year. If this happens the doctor may suggest doing further tests and may consider another operation.

WILL I NEED ANOTHER OPERATION?

It is also accepted that a bypass does not last forever, although with improved techniques they do now last for longer. Most people can expect a bypass to last for around ten to fifteen years, but some may find they need another bypass sooner than this. Greta, for example, whose blocked and furred arteries are a result of diabetes, was told she needed another within just five years.

John, who has high cholesterol levels, also needed another bypass five years after his first one. He says: 'Six months after my first heart surgery I thought: I'm struggling, I'm getting a bit breathless, so I went to the hospital and said, "I don't feel right. I'm getting chest pain like a steel band around my chest, squeezing." They didn't take much notice to start with but a year after the operation I went back for another angiogram to see if I could get my HGV licence back and they said that out of the four bypasses two were blocked, one was becoming blocked and they couldn't find the fourth one. Basically they said, "You're sick but you're not sick enough; come back when you are." '

You are likely to be very disappointed if you find that having surgery has not completely solved your problem and even more alarmed if you are told that you need a further operation. 'When they told me I needed a second bypass,' says John, 'the tears started streaming down my face. I knew it was the only option and I knew what to expect, but I was still upset.' It also has to be admitted that subsequent bypasses are not usually as successful as first ones, although they can still make a significant difference.

In this situation it is important to try to maintain a positive outlook. You may find that it helps to put into practice some of the self-help angina management techniques described in Chapter 2. Alternatively, you might like to think about exploring some complementary therapies such as those discussed in Chapter 10.

SUPPORT AND REHABILITATION

If you have had any of these procedures you may well find that you are not offered rehabilitation automatically. If this is the case, or if you feel that the rehabilitation programme on offer does not meet your needs fully, or simply if you are not a joiner, you can devise your own programme.

Exactly what you include in a self-devised programme will vary according to your individual needs. The advice given in the rest of the book should give you some ideas. If you have a partner you will benefit from involving him or her, and you are more likely to succeed in sticking to a new diet or exercise regime if your partner understands what you are trying to achieve and supports you. He or she may also benefit in their own right.

It's a good idea to check with your doctor or the physiotherapist at the hospital to make sure you are fit to exercise and to get some tips on the amount and intensity you should be aiming for. The heart charities and local support groups may also be able to help you with leaflets and advice on diet, exercise, risk factors and so on.

Paul describes how he devised his own fitness programme: 'I made a positive effort to create a new beginning. The consultant was very inspiring. He's a runner himself. When I asked what my chances of running again were, he said, "Why not? But you ought to lose a bit of weight first." I was then 12½ stone. He put me on to the physiotherapist who suggested I started to walk three or four miles briskly. She said once I'd got up to four miles I could begin to walk and run. Eight weeks later I'd got up to ten miles most days. Three months after the operation I did a Fun Run for a charity: three miles in 25 minutes. I can honestly say I've never looked back.'

Should you decide to devise your own programme the checklist below may help you get started:

- Do you have accurate information about your condition and the way it is to be managed medically and have you understood it? What do you intend to do to find out more (e.g. get hold of a book, talk to your doctor, contact a heart support group, heart charity and so on)?
- Do you understand what heart disease risk factors apply to you? What might you do to reduce your risks?
- Are you aware of who you should you contact and what you should do if you develop any medical problems?
- What treatment options are there if you are anxious or depressed e.g. anti-depressant drugs, counselling and so on? Can your partner attend any counselling sessions? You may also like to get hold of some self-help books on dealing with stress, anxiety and/or depression.
- Who can you ask for advice on work, stopping smoking, losing weight, stress management and so on? The cardiac rehabilitation team at your local hospital may be able to help (some have special helplines), or you could consider ringing an information line, such as the one run by the UK's British Heart Foundation (see Useful Addresses). It is manned by trained cardiac nurses who can answer most of your questions.
- Is there anywhere you can obtain an exercise test to determine your fitness to undertake an exercise programme? This may be a formal treadmill test or a simple walking assessment. Ask your doctor or the physiotherapist at the hospital.
- What sort of exercise should you do? Is there a group you can attend if you wish? What can you do at home? As with someone who has had a heart attack, a support group (see page 126) can often help restore your optimism and give practical advice on things you are finding difficult.

CHAPTER 6

LOOKING AT YOUR LIFESTYLE

'Looking back, well I suppose it had to happen sooner or later. I had all the background history of a wrong way of living. A wrong diet, a stressful occupation, I was a heavy smoker and took little or no exercise. My heredity was none too good. My sister died at 51 from a massive heart attack and my father had his first stroke at 60.'

LEN

'For it is a Secret both of Nature and State that it is safer to change Many things than one. Examine thy customs of Diet, Sleep, Exercise ... and the like.'

ELIZABETHAN WRITER AND PHILOSOPHER FRANCIS BACON, ESSAYS OR COUNSELS CIVIL AND MORAL, 1595

LEARNING ABOUT RISK FACTORS

It is natural if you've been diagnosed with heart disease to wonder, 'Why me?' With any illness doctors studying patterns of disease try to assess people's chance of contracting it by examining what are known as risk factors. These are aspects of lifestyle, together with physical and sometimes mental traits which in studies of large numbers of people are consistently associated with a particular disease. The more risk factors you have the higher your risk of developing that disease.

Useful though it is to examine your risk factors it is important not to become obsessed with the idea of risk. Remember that when scientists talk about risk they are usually referring to large groups of people not you as an individual and bear in mind that it is virtually impossible to point to one single factor and say that this is the culprit.

Howard, who had a heart bypass after suffering for years with angina, was able to identify two particular risk factors: 'You do wonder, how is it that this has happened? I'm a very active person –

I still only weigh 9½ stone – so I was quite shocked when I developed heart disease. I used to play tennis and football and I walked and as a teacher I was always rushing around. But, when I really thought about it I realized that – probably because I didn't have to watch my weight – I was for decades totally unaware of my diet. When I told the consultant what I ate he said I had to cut back very heavily on my diet: no cakes, biscuits or fat at all. The other factor was that my father died of heart problems aged 50, so I saw something reflected there.'

Heart disease is what experts call a multi-factorial disease. This means that many different factors are involved in its development. Different ones apply to different people, and usually it is a combination of more than one that does the damage. Many, as we shall see, we can change for the better, but some risk factors are not within our control.

UNCONTROLLABLE RISKS

AGE

One of the main reasons there is so much heart disease in twentieth-century developed countries is quite simply because we are all living longer. The process of atherosclerosis takes a long time to develop and our bodies becomes less able to repair damage as we get older. Although you cannot do anything about the advancing years, you can make sure you are as healthy as possible for your age by watching your diet, staying physically active and so on.

GENDER

Between the ages of 35 and 44 men are six times more likely to sustain a heart attack than women. But one in nine women between 45 and 64 have heart disease and after the age of 65 women are as likely to suffer from heart disease as men. Being a woman can alter the statistical risk of controllable factors, such as smoking and alcohol (see Chapter 6), and research has also shown that diagnosis and treatment of women with heart disease can vary from that of men. Factors with special relevance to women, or which only affect women, such as pregnancy and the menopause, are looked at in detail in Chapter 9.

FAMILY HISTORY

It has long been known that some types of heart disease run in families. People from families with a history of **familial hyperlipidaemia** (sometimes also called hypercholesterolaemia), in which there are raised levels of cholesterol, are at risk of developing heart disease early – even in the absence of other risk factors like high blood pressure and smoking. Gene hunters have tracked down the gene which causes the abnormality in cholesterol handling and it is now possible to have a blood test to check your cholesterol and to see if you are at risk if FH runs in your family.

Even without this condition a tendency towards atherosclerosis and heart disease seems to run in some families. It's still not known exactly why, but there are some clues. In the past few years research has suggested that there may be genetic differences in the way our bodies handle fat. Another contributory factor may be high blood pressure, which also frequently runs in families. Research is trying to track down possible culprits in our genetic blueprint. A possible candidate is a gene known as angiotensinogen; this triggers production of a hormone, angiotensin, which is involved in the control of blood pressure.

Because heart disease is so common, most of us can identify family members who have had it, especially when they became elderly. One clue that there may be a more significant hereditary factor is if several members of your family have had a heart attack or suffered heart problems at a much younger age than usual (under 55 for female relatives and under 50 for male relatives).

Should you suspect that this is the case in your family, you can draw up a family tree going back two or three generations and mark the members who suffered from heart disease. Your doctor may suggest that you go for genetic counselling. If it does turn out that you have a history of heart disease you will need to be especially vigilant to keep other risk factors under control.

If you or your family come from India, Bangladesh, Pakistan or Sri Lanka, and especially if you are a woman, you have a higher risk of developing heart disease. It is not known exactly why south Asians are at a higher risk, although it may be partly related to diet and partly to problems in regulating the hormone insulin (insulin resistance). Significantly, people who have moved to the UK from south Asia tend to develop heart disease more quickly than their relatives who have remained in south Asia, which strongly suggests that lifestyle factors, such as decreased activity, play an important part. African-Caribbeans have been shown to have a higher than average risk of developing high blood pressure, again possibly as a result of diet, although there may well be other factors involved.

The important thing to bear in mind with such uncontrollable risk factors is to do what you can to combat controllable risk factors (as explained in the second part of this chapter) and, if you develop heart disease, to take full advantage of the treatment and rehabilitation options on offer.

DIABETES

Diabetes occurs when the body is unable to produce or respond properly to insulin, which helps the body to use blood sugar to produce energy. Diabetes has long been known to have damaging effects on the cardiovascular system, producing abnormalities in blood fats that may speed the development of atherosclerosis and also affecting cholesterol and triglyceride levels, so people with diabetes are more likely to develop heart disease.

Some experts now argue that a key factor in diabetes is a phenomenon known as **insulin resistance**, in which the insulin receptors on their cells are unable to respond to insulin. Insulin resistance can affect people without diabetes as well as those with it. These experts believe insulin resistance may be part of a wider syndrome that involves other risk factors such as obesity, hyperlipidaemia (high blood fats) and high blood pressure.

Diabetes is more common in women than men, and while it raises the risk of heart disease and heart attacks for both sexes, the risk seems to be even higher in diabetic women. The combination of smoking and diabetes is particularly hazardous, according to Graham Jackson, consultant cardiologist at London's Guy's Hospital. This may be because women with diabetes tend to have lower levels of beneficial HDL cholesterol than men, and smoking lowers HDL.

If you have diabetes you can help control its effects by paying attention to your diet, taking regular exercise, controlling your weight and taking any drugs or insulin prescribed by your doctor.

Although it is important for all of us to do all we can to lower the major risk factors for heart disease, once you have done so try to keep a sense of proportion. Remember that heart disease is a disease not a punishment. Blaming yourself or feeling guilty or inadequate for developing it is not useful and may increase feelings of helplessness which can be damaging to self-esteem and confidence and may even impede recovery.

TAKING CONTROL

Having looked at 'in-built' factors that may increase the risk of heart disease, there are also aspects of health or lifestyle which have in many studies been linked with heart disease. One of the most positive measures you can take is to look at your own lifestyle and work out ways in which you can change it for the better. When thinking about the sort of changes you need to make the advice given by Francis Bacon at the beginning of this chapter is hard to beat.

Knowing your personal risk factors for heart disease and working out ways in which you can moderate them can not only increase the fitness of your heart and blood vessels but can also help you to make more sense of your condition and give you a feeling of being more in control.

Some risk factors explored here are now more or less universally accepted as having an important part to play in the development of heart disease; others do not appear to contribute to heart problems in quite the same clear-cut way. They may seem to bump up the risk of heart problems by acting in partnership with other established risk factors or cause damage in ways that are not entirely understood.

SMOKING

One of the most positive things you can do – and must do if you have been told you should have coronary surgery – is to give up smoking. A smoker under 50, whether a man or woman, is five times at risk from developing heart disease. Not just that, but if you smoke you are more likely to die from heart disease. In the UK alone just under a quarter of the men who die of coronary heart disease and just over a tenth of women do so because they smoke. In fact, it is estimated about half the 100,000 smoking-linked deaths each year are a result of arterial disease.

For women, smoking is an added hazard. Cigarette smoke reduces levels of 'good' HDL cholesterol, but in women it also lowers levels of oestrogen, the female sex hormone which is thought to have a protective effect on the arteries. In the Nurses' Health Study carried out in the USA women who smoke between just one and four cigarettes a day have double the risk of developing heart disease, while women who smoke 5–15 cigarettes a day have three times the risk. If you smoke more than 20 cigarettes a day your risk of a heart attack could be five times that of someone who doesn't smoke. Smoking also multiplies the dangers of other risk factors in women. Women who have diabetes, high blood cholesterol or who take the contraceptive Pill are all more likely to develop heart disease if they smoke too.

The good news is that if you stop smoking, no matter how long you have been a smoker, your risk of heart disease starts to go down. Within three years of giving up, your risk of dying is almost the same as for someone who has never smoked.

Helping yourself quit

There is no absolutely foolproof way to give up, but there are several strategies and aids you can use to help yourself. Some people find the motivation from books, inspirational individuals, videos, or from the knowledge that quitting will improve their health and well-being. If you have tried to give up in the past and failed, the fact that you have developed heart disease is proof of the damage that it is doing to your health and may just give you the extra willpower you need this time.

Gill, who quit when she was told she needed a heart bypass operation, says, 'I think sheer terror was the motivation. I'd tried before with nicotine patches and all sorts of things but they didn't work basically because I didn't want to stop. When I went to the hospital they said that if I carried on smoking I'd need another bypass in five years' time. I went home, smoked a packet of cigarettes and then gave up just like that. I haven't smoked since. I do still get the urge sometimes but I never succumb.'

Some of the methods advised by various organizations and publications include:

- Do you always light up after a meal, when you pick up the telephone, when relaxing, with a drink, at work? Once you have identified the circumstances in which you reach for a cigarette try to change your routine slightly or substitute some other activity.

- Learn better ways of managing stress (see page 101). People often light up to help them through situations which they find stressful such as meeting someone new, making a difficult phone call, having to meet a deadline and so on. Use other techniques such as breathing or relaxation methods to help you over stressful situations.
- Pay attention to diet. Heavy smokers often prefer to light up rather than eating and women especially often use cigarettes to control weight. Eating a balanced healthy diet and sticking to regular mealtimes will help curb the urge to nibble between meals. Incidentally, when you do give up avoid substituting sweets for cigarettes or you will put on weight.
- Cut down on caffeine. Smokers often consume a lot of caffeine in the form of tea, coffee or soft drinks. Too much caffeine tends to increase anxiety, nervousness and symptoms such as shakiness and tremor, which may in turn may lead to the urge to light up a cigarette in an attempt to calm down.
- Get support. Give up with your partner, a friend or join a stop-smoking group. In the UK many family doctors run such groups as part of their health education programmes. Alternatively join a group organized by a stop-smoking organization or individual.
- Save the money you normally spend on cigarettes and use it to buy yourself something you would like such as a new outfit, some sportswear or equipment, membership to a gym, a holiday or put it into a savings plan.

If you feel you could do with extra help ask your doctor about aids such as nicotine patches, gum and so on. Some ex-smokers have quit with the aid of complementary therapies ranging from hypnotherapy to acupuncture. These can act as valuable boosters to your motivation.

At the end of the day only you can stop smoking, so find the way that suits you. Most of the stop-smoking organizations such as the British charity Quit argue that it is more effective to set a day and then give up. However, some people find that it suits them better to cut down gradually over several weeks. There is no one right way for everyone, so use whatever method works for you. And if at first you don't succeed – try again.

HIGH BLOOD PRESSURE (HYPERTENSION)

Doctors still do not know exactly why some people develop high blood pressure, medically known as **hypertension**, although in some cases it does seem to run in families. People of African-Caribbean origin are also more at risk of high blood pressure. Obesity increases blood pressure, too, and this is obviously linked to your diet – salt, for instance, has been strongly implicated in raising blood pressure (see Chapter 7). Heavy drinking can also push up blood pressure. Finally high blood pressure can be caused by other medical conditions such as thyroid problems, diabetes and other hormonal imbalances, as well as liver or kidney disease.

The risk of coronary heart disease is linked to the level of your blood pressure. If you have high blood pressure and also smoke, are overweight, have diabetes or high blood cholesterol levels your risk of a heart attack (or stroke) increases even more. Insidiously high blood pressure is often silent. People usually do not realize they have it until a chance blood pressure reading by the doctor reveals the problem.

The British Heart Foundation says that for each 5mmHg reduction in blood pressure your risk of heart disease drops by around 16 per cent, so it is well worth your while taking all the steps you can to reduce your blood pressure. A combination of drug treatment and self-help can reduce blood pressure to normal.

Blood pressure tends to rise slightly as we get older and the arteries naturally become stiffer and less elastic. Raised blood pressure is even more strongly linked to the risk of developing heart disease in women. According to the American Heart Association, nearly half of all women in the US have high blood pressure and over the age of 75 women are more likely to develop high blood pressure than men. As with men, treating severely raised blood pressure seems to help reduce the risk, but what doctors are not so certain about as yet is whether treating women with only mild high blood pressure is beneficial. Taking drugs to lower mild hypertension does, however, seem to reduce the incidence of heart disease linked to a condition called **isolated systolic hypertension** (in which the upper figure of the blood pressure is raised), which affects women more than men.

What is blood pressure?

Blood pressure is the pressure exerted by the flow of blood through the body's main arteries. Blood pressure is created by a combination of two factors: the contraction of the heart as it pumps blood into the arteries and by the resistance of the body's smaller arteries or arterioles.

Blood pressure is measured by recording two measurements. The **systolic pressure** is the pressure of the blood flow when the heart contracts. The **diastolic pressure** is the pressure between heart beats. Blood pressure is usually measured using an instrument called a sphygmomanometer, which consists of a cuff with an air bladder connected to a tube and a bulb for pumping air into the bladder. A mercury gauge indicates pressure.

The effects of high blood pressure
In an adult a blood pressure of 140/80 or lower is not anything to worry about. Blood pressure tends to rise and fall over the course of the day and in response to circumstances such as exercise, stress and sleep. If blood pressure is consistently raised, especially if it reaches levels of 160/95 or greater it can damage the arteries, making them more vulnerable to atherosclerosis. High blood pressure means that the heart is working harder than usual. Over time this causes the heart to enlarge and this in turn may lead to heart failure. High blood pressure is also linked to stroke and kidney failure.

Medical ways to control blood pressure
Drugs used to lower blood pressure include diuretics to rid the body of excess fluids and salt; beta-blockers to reduce the heart rate and the work of the heart; vasodilators to relax and widen the walls of the blood vessels; ACE inhibitors, which interfere with a chemical that causes the smaller arteries to constrict; and calcium antagonists that reduce the heart rate and relax blood vessels. You will find more details of these drugs in Chapter 4.

Self-help ways to lower your blood pressure
The three most important ways you can lower your blood pressure are to pay attention to your diet, to take more exercise and to lose weight if you need to. You will find more on all these in Chapter 7. There is also some evidence that deep relaxation or meditation can lower blood pressure (see Chapter 10). The combined contraceptive Pill raises blood pressure in some women, so if you are, or intend to be, on the Pill, this is something you should discuss with your doctor.

Should you monitor your own blood pressure?
Various blood pressure monitors are available commercially and you may be tempted to buy one to keep a check on your blood pressure yourself. Before you do so it is worth considering a few points. First, some of the devices on the market are unreliable and some are costly. Secondly, blood pressure can vary from hour to hour and day to day: an isolated high reading can be worrying even though it is actually insignificant. Blood pressure is just one of a number of risk factors and becoming too obsessed with one particular factor is less useful than paying attention to your overall lifestyle. Thirdly, taking an accurate blood pressure reading is a skilled procedure, which is difficult for those who aren't medically trained.

The British Heart Foundation says: 'Generally speaking, measurement of blood pressure is best left to the professional, unless you have been advised to monitor your own blood pressure and have been instructed on how to do it by your doctor.'

RAISED LEVELS OF BLOOD FATS (HYPERLIPIDAEMIA)

The chemistry of fats in the blood stream has attracted a good deal of research and debate over the years. High levels of blood fats, or **lipids**, are associated with a higher risk of heart disease. The lipids story, however, is rather more complicated than that simple statement might suggest as there are several different types of blood fats and each is associated with a different risk of heart disease. The main message to take on board is that you can affect levels of blood fats by watching what you eat. A diet low in saturated animal fats and high in fruit and vegetables will help to ensure that your lipids remain in a desirable balance. Exercise also seems to have a favourable effect on blood fats (see Chapter 7).

The cholesterol question
The type of lipid everyone has heard of in connection with heart disease is **cholesterol**. According to the British Heart Foundation, lowering blood cholesterol levels by just 1 per cent can reduce your risk of heart disease by 2–3 per cent.

Cholesterol is a waxy substance produced mainly in the body by the liver but also present in certain foods, such as eggs, prawns and offal. As explained in Chapter 1 (see page 16), there is 'good'

HDL cholesterol and 'bad' LDL cholesterol. A certain amount of cholesterol is needed by the body to help build cell membranes, but too much LDL cholesterol can be harmful. Cholesterol forms a large part of the plaques found in atherosclerosis and numerous studies have shown that a high cholesterol level can accelerate the process of atherosclerosis.

Several factors can influence cholesterol levels. These include your age (high cholesterol may be more common as you get older); your family history (a tendency towards high cholesterol runs in some families); and diet (certain foods have a cholesterol-promoting and others a cholesterol-lowering effect). Overweight also increases blood cholesterol in some people. The cholesterol story may also be rather different for men and women and research is at present going on to try to identify the healthiest cholesterol levels for women. In the meantime, given that most people consume too much saturated fat, it still pays to follow the dietary guidelines outlined in Chapter 7.

Triglycerides

Many people with heart disease have high levels of a type of blood fat called triglyceride. According to the American Heart Association, 'High triglycerides are especially dangerous in people who smoke or have a strong family history of heart disease. In a person with no other risk factors and no family history, a high triglyceride level is less cause for concern than high blood cholesterol.'

Scientists still have a great deal to find out about triglycerides. High levels are not on the whole thought to be directly involved in furring of the arteries, as is the case with cholesterol, but high triglyceride levels when combined with low levels of HDL and high levels of LDL cholesterol tend to speed up atherosclerosis.

Triglyceride levels tend to be raised in people who are obese or drink heavily, and also in people with diabetes – all separate risk factors for heart disease. High triglyceride levels have also been found in women taking the contraceptive Pill. Losing weight and reducing excessive alcohol consumption can often lower triglyceride levels.

High-density lipoproteins

Low levels of HDL, 'good' cholesterol, are also linked to atherosclerosis. It is thought that this is because HDL 'hoovers up' excess LDL cholesterol and takes it back to the liver where it can be disposed of.

Because the blood fats all work in harmony, low HDL levels tend to be associated with high triglyceride levels. Lack of exercise, overweight, high overall cholesterol and smoking are also linked to low levels of HDL. Increased exercise and a small alcohol intake can raise HDL levels.

MEASURING BLOOD FATS

The British and the Americans measure blood fats in different ways. In Britain they are measured in units of **millimoles per litre**, or **mmol/l**, of blood. In the UK a level of less than 0.9mmol/l of HDL is considered low, while a total cholesterol reading above 6.5mmol/l is considered too high. The British Heart Foundation recommends that people with levels exceeding 5mmol/l should eat a cholesterol-lowering diet, but points out that most Britons have levels higher than this. Triglyceride levels are considered to be raised if they are over 2.3mmol/l.

In America blood fat levels are expressed in **milligrams per deciliter**, or **mg/dl**, of blood. According to the American Heart Association, many US scientists believe that the ideal total cholesterol level for American adults is under 200mg/dl. An HDL level of less than 35mg/dl is low. A normal level of triglycerides is considered to be less than 200mg/dl.

Medication for high levels of blood fats

Various drugs are used to treat hyperlipidaemia. Most of them are designed to lower cholesterol in various ways. If diet alone does not lower your blood fat levels or if levels are especially high your doctor may prescribe lipid-lowering drugs or refer you to a specialist lipid clinic. Several types of drugs may be used, depending on your exact blood fat profile. These include drugs which bind to bile acids such as cholestyramine and colestipol, fibrates which are used when both cholesterol and triglyceride levels are raised, nicotinic acid (niacin) (although this is less often used in the UK) and acipimox, which is also used when both triglycerides and cholesterol are raised. Some of the most effective cholesterol-lowering drugs are those called statins.

Another drug called probucol is sometimes used to lower cholesterol and fish oil is sometimes prescribed to lower triglycerides. You'll find more detail about these drugs in Chapter 4.

Self-help ways to influence your blood fat levels
One of the most important ways you can lower your blood fat levels is to stop smoking. Cigarettes, as we have seen, boost levels of 'bad' LDL cholesterol. Other ways are to watch your diet and to take more exercise (see Chapter 7). There is also evidence that learning to relax or meditate may influence blood fat levels. For information on this, see Chapter 10.

Cholesterol testing kits
Much the same advice applies to home cholesterol-testing kits as applies to commercial blood pressure monitors. The interpretation of cholesterol levels is extremely complicated and many different factors come into play, and a high level in itself does not always mean that you are at excess risk of heart problems any more than a low one means that you will avoid them. Home testing kits give only crude measures of the level of your cholesterol. They may also be unreliable and a false reading can cause much anxiety. If you do have high cholesterol you should ideally be under the supervision of your doctor or specialist who can perform a more sophisticated analysis of your blood fats and explain what the implications are.

PHYSICAL INACTIVITY

Being inactive is now fairly well established as a risk factor for heart disease. Research carried out in New Zealand, Australia and the US show that between a quarter and a third of adults are not active enough, especially older men and women, while in the UK it is estimated that half the adult population don't lead active enough lives. A sedentary lifestyle is associated with higher levels of cholesterol and triglycerides, lower levels of 'good' HDL cholesterol and overweight.

Being reasonably active, by contrast, can actively protect against heart disease. A study carried out in the UK early in 1997 looking at the effects of increased physical activity on coronary heart disease predicted that 12,000 people's lives could be saved over 25 years simply by people becoming more active. If you need further convincing, consider these facts, all based on research:

- Regular activity helps reduce levels of LDL cholesterol, the 'bad' cholesterol that clogs the arteries, and increases levels of protective HDL cholesterol.
- Moderate activity is effective in lowering raised blood pressure – even without the use of drugs. Aerobic exercise can lower systolic and diastolic blood pressure by 5–10mm of mercury.
- Activity reduces the stickiness of small blood cells called platelets, involved in blood clotting. Since blood clots are one of the main triggers for heart attacks and strokes, this is beneficial.
- Activity helps the body use insulin more efficiently and helps combat rises in blood sugar. Diabetes is an independent risk factor for heart disease and people with insulin-dependent diabetes often find that embarking on a programme of regular moderate exercise helps reduce their need for insulin.
- Activity alters the body's metabolism and helps your body burn fat more efficiently. Regular exercise encourages the body to use fat for energy. This can help raise levels of beneficial HDL cholesterol.
- Activity increases the body's demands for energy and can help to control appetite, which can help you to stick to a diet more easily. Even if you don't need to lose weight the improved muscle tone exercise brings will help you look slimmer and trimmer.
- Activity helps combat depression and loss of confidence that are common after a diagnosis of heart disease or a heart attack. During exercise the body releases chemicals called endorphins which boost feelings of well-being.

Research shows that women are often even less physically active than men. According to a British Heart Foundation leaflet, *Women and Heart Disease*, few British women take enough exercise: 'They say they are "not sporty", shy, too overweight or lack the energy or time. They rarely have a job which is physically demanding and only 20 per cent go in for a vigorous sport like swimming, aerobics and dancing. Two-thirds of women of any age are so unfit they cannot walk 3 miles (less than 5km) on a gradual, 5 per cent slope without having to stop, and 49 per cent between the ages of 65 and 74 cannot keep up a normal walking pace on the flat.'

You will find advice on starting to becoming more active and on maintaining levels of activity in Chapter 7.

OVERWEIGHT

The US Framingham Heart Study put obesity third after age and blood fat levels as a risk factor for heart disease – higher than blood pressure or smoking.

The US Nurses' Health Study showed that 40 per cent of heart disease in women could be attributed to being overweight. According to the British Heart Foundation 44 per cent of UK men and 33 per cent of UK women weigh more than they should do but are not classified as obese; a further 15 per cent of men and 18 per cent of women are clinically obese, which means that their weight is a threat to their health.

The most effective way of finding out if you need to lose weight – apart from looking in the mirror – is to work out your **body mass index** or **BMI**, which is the relationship between your weight and your height. To do this take your weight in kilograms and divide it by the square of your height in metres. If the figure you come to is 30 or more you are obese. As an example, if you are 1.65m (5ft 5in) tall and weigh 60kg (9 stone 6lb):

1.65 x 1.65m = 2.72.   60 divided by 2.72 = 22.05.

Then compare your answer with the following table:

	Men	Women
underweight	20 or less	18.6 or less
acceptable	20.1–25	18.7–23.8
overweight	25.1–29.9	23.9–28.5
obese	30+	28.6+

In a paper published in the *British Medical Journal* in May 1997, a team led by Professor Gerald Shaper found that even men who are not technically overweight have a higher risk of developing coronary heart disease and the report suggests that a BMI of 22 is a healthy goal for the average middle-aged man.

Why does it matter if you are overweight? Well, according to the British Heart Foundation, your risk of dying of heart disease is virtually doubled if you are male and overweight and is even higher if you are a woman. Research shows that people who are overweight are more likely to suffer from angina and sudden death from a heart attack.

Doctors still do not know exactly why being overweight should have such devastating effects on the heart, though of course excess pounds increase the amount of work your heart has to do. In theory, though, this should not be such a big problem as the heart is designed to work hard. A more significant factor could be that overweight people are, as we have already seen, more likely to have high levels of LDL cholesterol and high blood pressure – both of which are independent risk factors for heart disease.

Again, weight seems to be even more significant for women, who would seem to be more at risk when they are only mildly overweight. The harsh fact is that if you are an overweight woman you are four times more likely to die of a heart attack then your slimmer sister.

There is now quite a lot of evidence to show that it is where you carry your fat rather than your absolute weight which is the key factor. Various studies have now found that people who have a round 'apple' shaped figure (typically men) and who store fat around their waist and upper body have a higher risk of heart disease than those with 'pear-shaped' figures (typically premenopausal women) in which fat is stored around the hips and thighs. The American Heart Association says that if you are a man your waist should not measure more than your hips and if you are a woman your waist should not measure more than 80 per cent of your hips.

You can do much to enhance your cardiovascular health simply by shedding those extra pounds. You could be advised to ask your doctor for help in losing weight and this may prove helpful, but it has to be said that not all doctors are terribly interested in diet and you may find that he or she just thrusts a duplicated diet sheet at you and expects you to get on with it. If you are extremely self-motivated you may be able to lose weight on your own simply by following such a diet sheet. However, many people find that it helps their motivation to follow a more organized programme, either by investing in a good diet book or joining a slimming group. You will find more advice on losing weight in Chapter 7.

ALCOHOL

On of the biggest controversies surrounding heart diesease relates to alcohol. Alcohol, and wine in particular, has been used medicinally since ancient times. In modern times, however, it has generally been thought until the past few years that alcohol was bad for people with heart disease. Thinking on this started to change when researchers began to investigate the rather startling paradox that people in France, Greece and other Mediterranean countries who drank wine actually had lower rates of heart disease.

Numerous studies have confirmed that people who drink small amounts of alcohol have lower rates of heart disease than those who drink no alcohol. Gradually the tide of opinion began to turn and today it is generally accepted that moderate amounts of alcohol can help protect against heart disease in men aged over 40 and women past the menopause.

So why include alcohol in a chapter dealing with risk factors? As with so many aspects of coronary heart disease, the alcohol story is far from simple. Alcohol is a drug and, like any drug, it has risks as well as benefits. Scientists are now trying to work out more precisely the point at which the risks of alcohol outweigh its benefits and there is currently a great deal of controversy about what level of consumption is desirable.

How much?

The UK government's current advice is that men should keep their consumption below 21 units of alcohol a week and women below 14 units a week. A unit is equal to half a pint of beer, a glass of wine or a single measure of spirits. However, it is generally agreed that these limits are somewhat arbitrary, as alcohol affects us all differently, depending on our individual constitution, and some people may experience damaging effects at much lower levels.

What is known is that high levels of alcohol (over 40 units for men) are linked to higher rates of heart disease. Epidemiologist Dr John Kemm, writing in the *British Medical Journal* in November 1993, points out that in most studies men who drink about 7 units a week have rates of heart disease that are close to the lowest, while higher risks of dying from any cause coincide with drinking more than 21 units a week.

The picture is even muddier where women are concerned.

Women's bodies deal differently with alcohol. It is well known, for instance, that women process alcohol less efficiently in the run-up to a period.

Which drink is best?

Another thorny question is which type of alcoholic drink is most beneficial and here the picture is even less clear. In an editorial published in the *British Medical Journal* in May 1996, statistician Dr Ian White cites the well-known observation that people who live in countries in which more wine is drunk have less risk of dying from heart disease, whereas the link is weaker or absent in countries in which beer or spirits are more popular. Over the past few years this has led to the suggestion that wine may be especially beneficial in protecting the heart against disease. Some experts argue that red wine has the edge because it contains more anti-oxidant chemicals, which zap free radicals, the harmful molecules which are involved in both furring of the arteries and heart disease. This idea needs to be treated with great caution as results are contradictory and there may be other factors at work, such as cultural patterns of drinking, diet or social class that could explain the difference in risk. In Mediterranean countries, for example, people tend to have a glass of wine with food, rather than binge on spirits, and their diet customarily includes olive oil rather than saturated fats and a much higher percentage of fruit and vegetables.

How might alcohol protect?

The precise mechanism by which alcohol may be cardio-protective is not fully understood. Anti-oxidants may have some part to play, but it is thought that the main beneficial effect may be due to the fact that it raises levels of 'good' HDL cholesterol. Some studies have also found that, in women, alcohol pushes up oestrogen levels in the blood, which has a protective effect on the heart. On the other hand, alcohol also raises blood pressure, triglyceride levels and can cause irregular heart beats.

Clearly more research is needed before there can be any firm conclusions about drinking. At present the consensus seems to be that by and large the optimum level of alcohol intake should be no more than 1–2 units a day. If your triglyceride levels are high, your doctor may advise reviewing your intake of alcohol and perhaps advise you to stop drinking altogether. It is also worth bearing in mind, if you are watching your weight, that alcohol of any kind is high in calories.

LINKS BETWEEN THE MIND AND THE BODY

In the past many doctors have tended to concentrate more on physical explanations for developing heart disease, such as high blood pressure, than psychological ones. Such an approach fails to take account of other less tangible risk factors which may also be important. As a result, a number of experts have begun to take a more holistic approach and to look more closely at risk factors involving both the mind and the body in an attempt to reach a better understanding of what causes heart disease.

THE ROLE OF STRESS

Most people – whether they have heart disease or not – would probably say if asked that stress is a major risk factor for heart disease, so it's rather surprising to discover that the experts by no means all agree. In fact, stress as such does not feature on the lists of the four most significant risk factors put out by either the British Heart Foundation or American Heart Association.

Nevertheless, over the years a large number of studies have found links between having heart disease, stressful life events and various other social factors that are often linked to stress such as having a demanding job in which you have little or no control, being poor, not having a supportive network of friends and relatives you can turn to and so on.

As with men the type of work women do is significant. The US Framingham study revealed that women in clerical jobs had a higher risk of having a heart attack. This could well be because of the nature of clerical jobs which involve a lot of routine tasks imposed by someone else – the typical high-demand/low-control equation that has been linked to an increased risk of heart disease in men.

Among stay-at-home women, according to the American Heart Association, the following factors are linked to an increased risk of having a heart attack:

- symptoms of tension and anxiety
- being lonely during the day

- having trouble falling asleep
- infrequent holidays
- the belief that you are prone to heart disease.

Despite the persistent belief that stress is a major cause of heart problems, no one has yet come up with a definitive explanation of how stress actually affects the heart and blood vessels. One explanation of the possible relationship between stress and heart disease is that people who perceive themselves to be under uncontrollable or unmanageable stress are more likely to reach for the cigarette packet, drink too much alcohol or comfort eat and gain weight – all of which *are* recognized risk factors for heart disease.

A group of Finnish researchers reporting in the *British Medical Journal* in 1996 have come up with another, more intriguing suggestion. The researchers found that some men with early signs of furring of the arteries (atherosclerosis) tended to have exaggerated rises in blood pressure and heart rate in response to stressful events. When these same men were exposed to high demands at work they had 46 per cent more progression of atherosclerosis than other men who did not react in this way. The researchers concluded that, in people whose cardiovascular systems already have a biological predisposition to react strongly towards stress – as evidenced by their rise in blood pressure and heart rate – and where those same people already have evidence of the early signs of heart disease, being exposed to stress may in some way contribute to further furring of the arteries.

The researchers' finding is important because it is a far cry from simply saying: too much stress equals heart disease. It is also an extremely encouraging finding for people with heart disease because it suggests that learning to manage your reactions to stress could make a very real and significant difference to the state of your arteries.

SELF-HELP STRESS MANAGEMENT

Stress management often forms an integral part of rehabilitation programmes laid on for people recovering from a heart attack or heart surgery. There are also various courses just on stress management run by local education authorities and private organizations. It is well worth checking these out.

SUGGESTIONS FOR DEALING WITH STRESS:

- Take regular exercise. Exercise helps dissipate stress hormones such as adrenalin which if left in the body can have an effect on the heart.
- Practise relaxation. Relaxation quietens the body physically and also induces calm alpha-waves in the brain which allow both body and mind to get the rest they need to recover from a period of stress.
- Make time for activities you enjoy. Working all the time may be harmful if you never allow yourself time to rest. Hobbies, sports, holidays and other activities you enjoy allow your body and mind a break from the stress of everyday life.
- Learn to be assertive. A major cause of stress is taking on too much and then being unable to cope with the demands made upon you. Many people feel unable to say 'No' for fear of offending or because they want other people to think well of them. Learn to say 'No' and stick to your decision.

When faced with a stressful event:
- Think about its likely course and what is likely to be demanded of you, then plan how to respond.
- Put the actions needed in order of priority and set yourself a time scale. Be realistic. Rushing things is a major cause of stress.
- Think about other ways of dealing with the stressful situation. Can you share or delegate some of the necessary action to other people?
- Share your feelings about the stressful situation with someone you trust. Don't be afraid to ask for support and help. There is no virtue in doing everything alone.
- After a stressful event take a break. Stressful situations are by their nature demanding so build in some recovery time.

But no matter how many courses you go to, at the end of the day it is up to you to change your reaction to stress. Howard describes how he made a real effort after his heart bypass to tackle his reaction to stress: 'I was very concerned about stress and tried not to let myself get worked up about things. If something was making me feel stressed I would force myself to withdraw from it. I just said "What's the point?" If I'm going to be late for a meeting I'm going to be late. I am very highly strung but I made a conscious effort. I surprise myself now by all things I used to do and committees I attended. I never said "No" to anything. Now I'm much more selective.' Reducing stress, however, does not mean withdrawing from all activities.

IS THERE A CORONARY PERSONALITY?

For several years now psychologists have been trying to determine whether there is such a thing as a cardiac-prone personality. In the 1970s US psychologists Friedman and Rosenman identified a clutch of traits they described as 'Type A personality' in their book *Type A Behaviour and Your Heart*. These traits were said to increase the risk of heart disease and included: excessive hard-driving behaviour, time urgency, job involvement, competitiveness, aggressiveness and hostility.

Over the past 20 years psychologists have been attempting to narrow down exactly which aspects of Type A behaviour might be most damaging to the heart and have identified hostility, and in particular a type of hostility described as 'expressed anger' – getting openly angry and irritated by everyday events and other people – as the main culprit. Some psychologists are now to trying to link this with what happens in the nervous system and blood vessels when someone is constantly angry. 'When expressed anger becomes habitual the person becomes chronically aroused,' points out Dr Mark McDermott, lecturer and researcher in health psychology at the University of East London. He explains how this might contribute to furring of the arteries: 'When the nervous system is aroused by anger fatty acids are released, some of which are converted in the liver into "bad" cholesterol (LDL). If you are always angry your body is repeatedly releasing fatty acids which may get converted to LDL. As people get older levels of "good" cholesterol fall, so the ability of the body to mop up LDL decreases. However, anger does not fall, with the result that the person is chronically awash with damaging LDL. A second effect is that hormones released by such arousal tend to inhibit cell repair. A third possible mechanism is that chronic arousal is linked to high blood pressure.' His questionnaire on page 119 may be helpful in identifying expressed anger.

Again, there are differences between women and men. While anger and hostility have been found to be significant factors in men, in women a higher risk of heart disease is linked to tension, anxiety, worry over money, and the inability to get away from everyday pressures and relax.

Although conventional cardiologists sometimes pooh-pooh such ideas, they do provide a convincing link between the environmental, psychological and physical factors found to be involved in heart disease. Taking steps to combat anger, anxiety and tension with relaxation or meditation (see Chapters 9 and 11) could well make a difference to your risk of heart disease.

KEEPING A SENSE OF PERSPECTIVE

Having said all this, it is important to keep stress, anger and other psychological factors in perspective, as Professor Bob Lewin points out. Professor Lewin claims that the belief that stress is harmful can be detrimental to people recovering from heart disease because it may cause them to underplay the real physical risk factors they should do something about.

He cites a piece of research in which people who had had a heart attack were asked what they thought caused it: 'Most said psychological factors such as stress, worry and hard work. Even after a rehabilitation programme in which they were taught about risk factors, 80 per cent still said stress, worry and hard work. When they were asked which were the most damaging, they said stress, worry and hard work plus smoking. When asked which they would find most difficult to cope with, the biological risk factors were of no consequence – it was things which they felt they couldn't control, in other words stress, worry and hard work. We need to try to get people to put risk factors in the right order.'

Clive, who had heart failure and had angioplasty following a heart attack, is a good example of this way of thinking. He says: 'I'm a typical Type A and I wish I wasn't. If I wasn't so pushy I wouldn't have had heart failure. I should have learnt to relax more.' Later in our conversation Clive admitted that his idea of a good time was to go out with his friends and drink 12 pints of beer every night. He added: 'I was five stone overweight when I had my heart attack. I used to have a fried breakfast every day.' Was it the stress, his unhealthy lifestyle or a combination of both that caused his heart disease?

CHAPTER 7

EXERCISE AND DIET

*'I cook with olive oil and I use low-fat products. I don't fry
and I don't eat red meat – only chicken. I always used to
eat a lot of rice and pasta anyway so that hasn't changed.
I now use skimmed milk in tea and cooking. I don't take
sugar in my tea and I don't use salt. But other than that
I haven't changed that much.'*

CAROLYN

'I walk for half an hour a day and I swim. I really enjoy it.'

GILL

IF YOU GOT THIS FAR you will already be well aware of the benefits
for people with heart disease of exercising and eating a healthy
diet. These two factors are both such important aspects of a
healthy lifestyle that it is certainly worth being armed with as
much information as you can. This chapter contains detailed
information on diet and exercise based on the latest thinking. It
also contains tips designed to help you stay motivated so you
continue to stick with your healthy living plan. It is often one
thing to make changes in your lifestyle after a diagnosis of heart
disease or as part of a rehabilitation programme following a heart
attack or surgical procedure, and another to maintain them once
the first flush of enthusiasm has faded.

BECOMING MORE ACTIVE

If you have been diagnosed with heart disease or have had a heart
attack, it is important to build up levels of activity gradually and
to respect your own limits. You may be tempted to try to prove to
the world that you are fit. This is almost certainly unwise, as Gill,
who had a heart bypass when she was 51, points out: 'At first I
tried to do too much. I was getting very tired and had to cut back.
Now I'm more moderate in what I do. I find swimming is very
good and very therapeutic. So too is very gentle exercise, like
easing my shoulders back and lots and lots of walking. Every day
before I do anything else I walk for half an hour.'

Jim, who took up running after a triple bypass, comments: 'I run two to three miles most mornings. It takes about half an hour. I don't push myself, I take it at my own pace. Lots of people run when I do, first thing in the morning. They all come bounding past me, but I don't mind.'

The most beneficial kind of activity for the heart is aerobic, i.e. activity that is vigorous enough to make you slightly breathless. For a long time the expert advice on exercise has been to do a high-intensity aerobic activity such as aerobics, jogging, running, swimming, cycling or sports such as tennis or football, three times a week. Recent research suggests, however, that modest levels of low-intensity activity can be just as beneficial – provided it is done regularly.

In the UK many experts now recommend undertaking moderate physical activity for at least 30 minutes five times a week. This can be divided into shorter spells of 10–15 minutes at a time. Walking, which is both moderate and aerobic, is one of the best forms of exercise and is something the whole family can enjoy. Even if you have never enjoyed walking in the past it is worth trying to do more now. If you don't especially enjoy walking try to make it part of your daily life, for example by walking short distances to work or to the shops.

Vary your route to avoid boredom, try to include a walk around the park, along a river bank or head out for a local beauty spot. Start at a slow pace and gradually build up your speed and distance. Walk briskly but not so fast that you become exhausted. Pace yourself. This is especially important in the early days – remember that wherever you walk, you have to walk back. Other forms of moderate activity you might consider are dancing (any sort so long as it makes you slightly breathless), housework and gardening.

Some breathlessness is normal when you first start exercising, especially if you have always led a rather sedentary life or if you are overweight. It is usually a sign that you are unfit. A rule of thumb is that you should be able to talk while you are exercising. If you become so breathless that you are unable to talk you are working too hard. Listen to your body and be prepared to stop exercising if you feel unwell.

Certain activities are inadvisable if you have high uncontrolled blood pressure. These include anything that involves straining (so called isometric exercises) such as heavy lifting, including weightlifting, and high-intensity aerobic exercise. If your blood pressure is being controlled by drugs walking, jogging, cycling, swimming, tennis and low-resistance strength training should be safe. If your blood pressure is not controlled by drugs stick to lower-intensity activities such as moderate walking and golf.

STOP EXERCISING IF:

- You experience chest pain or pain that spreads to arms, jaws, back or abdomen
- You feel dizzy or light-headed
- You feel tired or generally unwell
- You are short of breath
- You feel nauseous
- You sweat more than usual
- You experience palpitations (an irregular or fast pulse rate)
- Your pulse rate does not diminish five minutes after you have stopped exercising

PACING YOURSELF

Always warm up for a few minutes before starting to exercise. Doing a few gentle stretches helps get your circulation going and helps avoid injury to your muscles and joints. A simple stretch routine will usually include arm stretches, shoulder stretches, calf stetches and thigh stretches. Regular stretching improves flexibility, which can help you to exercise more effectively. Wear something loose and comfortable that allows you to move freely when warming up. Stretch to the point where you feel a slight pull. Don't bounce or jerk. Stretching is also a good way to cool down when you have finished your exercise session.

Your resting pulse rate shows your overall level of fitness. To determine this take your pulse when you wake up in the morning. Count the beats for 15 seconds and multiply this by 4 to get the rate per minute. A resting pulse of over 100 beats a minute can be a sign of a heart problem. How soon your pulse returns to normal after exertion is another indication of how fit your heart is. It should return to normal after 5–6 minutes.

Very cold or hot weather conditions place an extra strain on your heart and high altitudes can be inadvisable because of lack of oxygen. Gill says: 'The whole family used to enjoy skiing. However, since my operation I find that if I go beyond 1500 metres I become breathless. I still haven't managed to ski again and I have to accept that I may never do so. However, I still enjoy being in the mountains and walking.'

STAYING ACTIVE

Regular continued activity is the key factor in maintaining a healthy heart. It may seem hard to set aside time for specific exercise, so try to include activity in your everyday routine: use the stairs rather than the lift, walk or cycle to work or part of the way to work.

It is always easier to feel enthusiastic about exercising if you have chosen an exercise that you enjoy. If you are a reluctant exerciser you may find it helps to 'disguise' exercise as something else that is fun or challenging. Enrolling in a class in Latin dance, for example, may be a better bet than taking a conventional aerobics class, which can be boring. Incidentally, if one of your chosen forms of exercise is playing a competitive sport such as tennis or golf, try to cultivate a spirit of friendly competition rather than an urge to win. Stay relaxed and concentrated and know your limits. If you must compete, try to beat your own previous performance rather than your opponent.

It is often possible to make extra time for exercise by making very simple changes in your lifestyle. Could you get up half an hour earlier, for example, so you can fit in a brisk walk before breakfast? Could you do some exercise in your lunch hour? Is it possible to fit in a swim, a dance class or a run on the way home from work? Look out for evening exercise sessions in your area. Many heart support groups hold follow-on exercise classes in the evening. If you intend to join a gym or go to a class, make it somewhere that is convenient to get to. If you have to travel for two hours to your exercise class the chances are you will not bother if you are feeling tired, or if it's cold or raining.

Weather is another factor to take into account. Tennis is a great aerobic activity but choose a club that has an indoor court or you won't be able to do it for most of the year. Safety is another consideration. It's not a good idea to go running in an unlit area of an inner city on dark winter evenings; better to join a local authority gym, confine your runs to daylight hours or invest in some exercise equipment you can use at home.

John, who helps run a post-rehabilitation exercise club held three nights a week in his local hospital, says, 'The exercise group started with 24 people, now we've got 124. I know full well if I didn't have the club they wouldn't exercise. It's not just the exercise, it's the camaraderie. We exercise, bounce feelings or thoughts off each other. It's better to do that than talk to a medical person.'

Clive agrees it is the camaraderie of others at the exercise group for cardiac patients he attends that keeps him going: 'It's good fun because we're all buddies together. You make friendships. If you don't come one week people want to know where you were.'

Gill, who took up going to the gym and swimming after being diagnosed with diabetes which is linked with a high risk of developing heart disease, is making exercise part of her daily routine: 'I do find it boring sometimes, but it is just something I accept that I do now, like cleaning my teeth. I work from home so I try to go in the afternoon when my brain isn't so alert anyway and then carry on working when I get back. I do feel better for it as well. I've noticed that I have more energy than I used to have and I can do more, so that keeps my motivation up as well.'

In some areas there are special fitness classes for people with heart problems. These may be organized by local heart support groups while others are offered as part of the local authority adult education programme. Once you have become relatively fit joining a gym may be a good idea. Many provide a fitness assessment before taking you on. Check that any gym you enrol with is supervised by qualified instructors and that staff are trained in CPR. It is important to be honest and tell the staff that you have heart disease. You should be taught how to take your pulse and monitor your progress.

DIET AND HEART DISEASE

Changing the way you eat, as we have already seen, is one of the best ways to help yourself. However, it can be hard to know exactly what to eat when even the experts seem to be confused. Scarcely a week passes without the newspapers telling us that some unsuspected ingredient is bad for our hearts or trumpeting some new wonder diet or food said to be vital for a healthy heart.

We've had the Mediterranean Diet, the Eskimo Diet and the Japanese Diet, to mention just a few.

A team at the Harvard School of Public Health writing in the *British Medical Journal* in 1997 sums up the current state of knowledge: 'A prudent approach for prevention of coronary disease... is to recommend a reduced intake of saturated fat, cholesterol and trans unsaturated fatty acids accompanied by an increased consumption of foods rich in fibre, including cereals, vegetables and fruit.' The guidelines on healthy eating given by the British Heart Foundation broadly conform to this advice.

FAT

The American Heart Association recommends keeping fat to less than 30 per cent of your total calories. Of this, saturated fatty acids (found in animal products, margarine and butter) should form less than 10 per cent of calories; polyunsaturated fatty acid intake (in the form of nut and seed oils and margarines) no more than 10 per cent, and monounsaturated fatty acids around 10–15 per cent. Trans fatty acids can develop from the hydrogenation, or solidification process, of oils. Some margarines, for example, are particularly high in trans fatty acids.

The best way to achieve the guidelines on fat is to cut down overall on the amount of fat and fatty foods in your diet. Red meat is a source of saturated fat. White meats such as chicken are a better bet, but it is still a good idea, says the American Heart Association, to confine your intake to no more than 6oz of lean meat or skinless poultry a day. You should also pay attention to cooking methods. Frying, especially in fat that has already been used once, releases free radicals which, as we have seen, are involved in atherosclerosis. Grill, steam, bake or stir-fry using very small amounts of an unsaturated oil such as olive oil or a nut oil rather than deep-frying. Choose skimmed milk or semi-skimmed milk and low-fat yoghurt and cheese.

New thinking about fat
We may be about to witness a sea-change in thinking about fat. In the past few years nutritionists have discovered that certain unsaturated fats called **trans fatty acids**, found in biscuits, margarine and cakes, may contribute to heart disease. As is so often the case, it is hard to disentangle cause and effect because

people who eat diets high in saturated fats and trans fatty acids often eat a diet which is also low in fibre, fruit and vegetables and oils such as olive oil which is high in mono-unsaturated fats and therefore protective against heart disease. As well as cutting down on red meat, cheese and butter it makes sense to eat fewer biscuits and processed food and replace these with more fruit and vegetables so as to reduce the number of trans fatty acids you consume.

An increasing amount of research shows that, while some kinds of fats are harmful to the arteries, others protect against atherosclerosis disease. Omega-3 fatty acids, a type of polyunsaturated fat found in oily fish such as herring, mackerel, swordfish and tuna, reduce the chances of further heart attacks in people who have already had one. There is also increasing evidence that linolenic acid, which is found in leafy vegetables, protect against heart disease. And a good deal of research is now being carried out into oleic acid, the fatty acid found in olive oil. In the past it was thought that monounsaturated fats were neutral in their effect on the blood vessels, but it is now thought that they may have a protective effect. The American Heart Association advises, 'Approximately 5–8 teaspoons of fats and oils per day may be used for cooking and in salad dressings and spreads.'

What about cholesterol?
Although most cholesterol is manufactured in the liver, some cholesterol comes from the diet. Cholesterol is found in organ meats such as liver, brains, kidneys, heart, sweetbreads and so on, so it makes sense to limit your consumption of these. It is also found in egg yolks. The AHA advises that you should limit consumption to 3–4 egg yolks a week, whether used alone or in cooking and baking (this includes bought cakes, biscuits and dishes that contain eggs).

FIBRE

An increasing number of studies have shown that a high-fibre intake can lower cholesterol levels. The type of fibre most significant in protecting against heart disease is the gluey, 'soluble' type found in the cell walls of pulses such as lentils, fruit such as apples and cereals like rye, barley and oats (this is the stuff that gives porridge its gooey, gelatinous consistency) rather than the husky bran variety found in wheat chaff.

'It's not known exactly how fibre exerts its protective effects,' explains Dr Ann Walker, senior lecturer in Human Nutrition at Reading University. 'There is the suggestion that short-chain fatty acids produced in the gut through fermentation inhibit the body's synthesis of LDL cholesterol. Another hypothesis is that cholesterol binds to fibre and is taken out of the body. An even more convincing argument is that some type of fibre bind to bile acids which would normally be converted into cholesterol.'

Good sources of fibre are wholegrain breads, cereals, rice and pasta. Fresh vegetables, dried fruit, nuts and baked beans also contain fibre. The American Heart Association advises eating six or more servings of breads, cereals or grains a day. It also advises trying main dishes featuring pasta, rice, beans and/or vegetables.

FRESH FRUIT AND VEGETABLES

Numerous studies have shown that people in countries with a plentiful intake of fruit and vegetables experience less heart disease. Fruit and vegetable intake in the UK averages about 200g a day compared to the Mediterranean average of 600–700g a day. Studies suggest that simply eating at least five portions of fruit and vegetables a day could reduce the number of deaths from heart disease by as much as 20–30 per cent.

Fruit and vegetables help keep the body's levels of sodium and potassium in balance, an important factor in controlling blood pressure, which is a risk factor for heart disease. Fruit and vegetables also contain a number of ingredients that actively protect the arteries against damage. As yet scientists do not know exactly what all these are. Some of the strongest candidates are nutrients known as anti-oxidants, which counteract the effects of free radicals, the harmful molecules involved in the oxidation of LDL cholesterol. In particular, vitamins C, E and beta-carotene, which is made into vitamin A in the body, are thought to be important to protect the heart. Collectively, these are known as the ACE vitamins.

Victamin C also works in conjunction with another protective nutrient, folic acid, which is a member of the B vitamin group found in green leafy vegetables, offal, eggs and wholegrain cereals.

As well as these known protective vitamins a lot of research is being carried out into other ingredients and compounds known as phytochemicals. A group of compounds called flavonoids, of which there are around 6000 found in a wide range of vegetables and vegetable-based products such as tea and red wine, may be especially important.

There are many ways to increase your fruit and vegetable intake. Experiment with vegetarian dishes. Slice some fresh fruit over your breakfast cereal or have a fresh fruit salad for breakfast. Check out exotic fruit and veg at the supermarket for variety.

SALT

A high intake of salt (sodium chloride) increases blood pressure. Some salt is necessary, of course, to maintain the body's sodium balance, but most of us could probably get by with much less salt than we consume – it is estimated that most people use 10–20 times more salt than is needed by the body.

Proof that cutting down on salt can help can make a significant difference to heart disease comes from Finland. Over the past few years both the Finnish food industry and individuals have been encouraged to use a special salt substitute instead of ordinary table salt, together with a whole range of other diet and lifestyle measures, and the incidence of deaths from heart disease has fallen by half.

Another huge study, known as the INTERSALT Project, was carried out in 30 different countries. Its results showed close links between the amount of salt consumed and blood pressure. The study also revealed a close relationship between salt intake and rising blood pressure as we get older. So if you have high blood pressure it makes sense to cut down on your salt intake.

The British Heart Foundation advises reducing your salt intake rather than always using a substitute, but cutting down on salt isn't simply a question of not reaching for the salt cellar when you eat your supper. A great deal of the salt we consume comes from convenience foods and snacks like crisps, peanuts and so on, so it's a good idea to cut down on these and substitute instead more fruit and vegetables, which help lower blood pressure too.

MAKING DIETARY CHANGES STICK

Changing your diet is often more effective if you make small changes gradually. Many people find it easier to stick to changes if they don't make them too extreme to start with. If you have a family to cater for this may be especially important, as you are likely to meet less opposition if all their favourite foods are not suddenly struck off the menu. On the other hand, US physician Dean Ornish argues, 'It is actually easier to motivate people to make big changes than small ones.' He claims that conventional dietary recommendations offer 'the worst of both worlds, because people feel deprived, but no better'. His hugely successful *Lifestyle Study* involved people following a strict vegetarian diet and making large reductions in dietary fat (see Chapter 10).

A lot will depend on your individual personality and what motivates you. Whichever path you choose to follow, the key to making dietary changes stick is to make them enjoyable. True, you may have to forgo a few foods that you enjoy now, but a huge number of foods are positively recommended – including the whole range of fruit and vegetables from all over the world, so you should never be short of delicious things to eat.

A feeling of deprivation saps good intentions so try to concentrate on what you *can* eat rather than constantly regretting what you can't, and give yourself time to get used to your new pattern of eating. You may well find, as Clive did, that once you have got used to eating more healthily you are no longer tempted by things that you used to enjoy, 'I loved fatty foods and I couldn't imagine giving up my fried breakfasts. Now if I walk past a hamburger joint and smell the onions it makes me feel sick. Twice a year I have a big plate of fish and chips and that's my treat. I don't feel I miss out.'

Making small changes by substituting one food for another is another way to ensure that you make changes with the minimum of upheaval. You will find that it gets easier as time goes on, as Gill observes, 'I used to cook with lots of butter. Now I use extra virgin olive oil, I buy low-fat cheeses and yoghurts, I use a low-salt product instead of salt, and I make a real effort when I go shopping to examine labels and think about what I'm buying. Both my husband and I feel better for it. At first it was a major deal, I bought lots of cook books and used to pore over them, but now it has become second nature.'

SHOULD I TAKE SUPPLEMENTS?

There's a good deal of controversy surrounding dietary supplements and it has to be said that many of the trials have contradictory results. Some conventional doctors and cardiologists are dubious about the benefits of supplementation and argue that we should be able to get all the nutrients we need from eating a well-balanced diet with plenty of fruit and vegetables, while others believe that supplements do help.

A number of studies do seem to indicate that certain supplements are beneficial in protecting against heart disease. The Cambridge Heart Antioxidant Study reported in 1996, for example, that people with furred arteries who took 400–800IU of vitamin E a day had a 77 per cent less risk of having a non-fatal heart attack, though there was no significant difference in their risk of dying of a heart attack. High levels of vitamin C also seem to reduce the chances of dying from heart disease, while a study from the US reported in the *American Journal of Clinical Nutrition* in 1996 showed that taking both vitamin C and vitamin E supplements decreased the risk of dying of heart disease by 53 per cent. Other trials either report no effect or, in the case of beta-carotene, show an increased risk of heart disease and lung cancer, especially in people who smoke.

A point worth making is that nutrients work in harmony, so it is very hard to prove that any one nutrient is protective. Vitamin C, for example, protects vitamin E, an oily vitamin, from oxidation. Similarly, folic acid works best in combination with vitamins B6 and B12. For this reason many experts recommend increasing your intake of fruit and vegetables generally rather than taking isolated supplements.

Dr Ann Walker, senior lecturer in Human Nutrition at Reading University is in favour of supplementation, but points out, 'It is impossible to get the amount of vitamin E needed to protect against heart disease from diet alone and it would be hard to get the 400 micrograms of folic acid that have been shown to protect against heart disease from diet alone.' She recommends taking a supplement of 500-600 IU vitamin E together with a mixed anti-oxidant supplement, adding, 'You have to be a bit careful with beta-carotene and use it only if it is mixed with other anti-oxidants and don't exceed 15mg a day.'

LOSING WEIGHT

You may find that following the advice given above helps you to lose weight, even without following a specific diet. However, if you need to lose more than a few pounds you will undoubtedly do so faster if you follow a proper calorie-controlled diet. The following tips are intended as general guidelines. For more detailed information seek the advice of your doctor, a dietitian or one of the slimming organizations.

- Take it gradually. Crash diets tend to work only for a short time and yo-yo dieting (taking weight off and then putting it on again) has in some studies been linked to a higher risk of heart disease. It is best to aim to lose a moderate 500g–1kg (approximately 1–2¼lb) a week.
- Go for starchy carbohydrate foods, fruit and vegetables and cut down on fats and fatty foods such as chips. Research shows that starchy foods help you to feel full, which means you are far less likely to nibble.
- Cut down on sugary foods, sweets, chocolate, cakes, biscuits, soft drinks and ice cream.
- Cut down on alcohol: it contains lots of calories.
- Don't be discouraged if weight loss slows down after the first couple of weeks. At first you will lose more because when you first start to diet your body generally loses weight more quickly.

OTHER WAYS TO HELP YOURSELF

Many experts working with people with heart disease comment that of all the lifestyle changes people try to make, losing weight seems to be the most difficult. For this reason it is a good idea to have a few tricks up your sleeve to keep up your motivation.

One thing which is certainly worth doing is to include exercise in your weight-loss plan. Physical activity is important in its own right, but exercise has other bonuses when it comes to effective weight loss. It pushes up your metabolism so that your body burns fat more effectively and helps to suppress appetite by raising levels of blood sugar which stops you feeling hungry.

As far as the heart is concerned, walking is one of the best forms of exercise. One study carried out a few years ago in the States showed that women can lose as much as 4in off their waist, hips and thighs in just two months, simply by walking for two hours a week.

Other things that can help are slimming with a friend (or your partner) or joining a group for extra encouragement and support.

CHAPTER 8

EMOTIONS, RELATIONSHIPS AND SEX

'Supporting a close friend or relative who has suffered from heart disease will help their recovery. However, in the process you may become more anxious about their health than they are themselves, and you may also take on the stress of new responsibilities at home such as gardening or bill payments.'

BRITISH HEART FOUNDATION BOOKLET, LIVING WITH HEART DISEASE

'Here had been this big strong man and all of a sudden he was like a child. It upset both of us. I had to learn to be the strong one; he had to learn to be vulnerable.'

LINDA

HEART DISEASE DOES NOT JUST AFFECT you physically. It also involves changes in your relationships with the people around you and may, as we have already seen, uncover a whole welter of confusing emotions. In many ways it's easier and less threatening to deal with the physical aspects of life such as paying attention to what you eat and exercising than it is to confront these difficult emotions. Men sometimes find this even harder than women.

DIFFERENT EMOTIONS

DENIAL

Some people react to the knowledge that they have heart disease by putting on a brave face, underplaying what has happened to them, refusing to acknowledge that there is anything wrong or being falsely optimistic. Psychologists refer to this type of reaction as denial.

Denial is the mind's way of coping with the initial shock of any adverse event, which is why it is often common immediately after people have had a heart attack. 'When I started to get all these strange symptoms I half thought that there was something wrong with my heart,' Gill says. 'When I went to the doctor I joked that something was wrong with my heart and in the office a few times when I came over strange I said I think I'm going to snuff it, but at the same time I didn't really believe it.'

Clive says: 'With angina, psychologically you are fighting to say that it's not there. It's important to me to deny it, because otherwise I get very paranoid and frightened.' As Clive points out denial can be a way of refusing to let an illness get the better of you. It is only if you are finding it difficult to take medical advice that this can become more problematic.

ANXIETY AND PANIC

When you are anxious your mind races, you are dominated by fearful thoughts, you feel physically tense and experience symptoms such as diarrhoea and shaking. You may sleep badly. People who are anxious tend to feel worse in the evening, whereas people who are depressed often feel most miserable in the morning. In both anxiety and depression you may experience headaches and other aches and pain, and attribute these to your heart. You may find it difficult to concentrate and feel tired as a result of using nervous energy. A fear of recurrence may be worsened by real physical symptoms such as palpitations. Bear in mind that while these may be related to your heart, such symptoms are also a result of anxiety.

Panic is an extreme form of anxiety. Many people experience panic attacks after a diagnosis of heart disease or a heart attack. They can be particularly alarming because the symptoms may be confused with having a heart attack.

Linda describes Len's reaction after he came home following a bypass: 'The panic attacks he experienced in those first weeks were the worst to cope with because you could never be sure if the pain was due to a real malfunction or merely a result of his anxiety. When they were really bad he believed them to be the onset of a heart attack, which increased his tension and tightening of the muscles causing further pain, so that in the end his fear almost became reality.'

'At these times nothing I could say or do seemed to help and it was only by taking him to the nearest hospital that it was possible to allay those fears. Once they had placed him on an ECG machine and told him everything was functioning well, the fear and tension were relieved and we were able to carry on until the next time.'

Your doctor or a cardiac nurse will often be able to help alleviate your fears by giving you accurate facts about your illness. Jo Partington, a British Heart Foundation nurse in Harrogate, says: 'Patients are often petrified when they go home after a heart attack. They believe their heart is damaged beyond repair. I make sure they understand that although the heart has been damaged it heals up. Often this is enough to help them feel better.'

Sometimes dealing with panic is simply a matter of time. As well as having accurate facts about your illness it helps to recognize what the signs of a heart attack are so you can distinguish between them and panic. Using a relaxation technique such as the one described in Chapter 10 or listening to a relaxation tape can also be helpful.

ANGER

Some people react to all their confused feelings by becoming angry and irritable. Anger is often much easier to deal with than fear or depression. This anger may be directed at hospital staff, the doctor, your partner, children, friends, colleagues or simply life in general.

If you find you are habitually angry it can help to spend some time thinking about how you normally deal with anger and then work out some more effective ways of coping with it. Psychologists who have studied anger have found that people who are habitually at odds with the world often become angry because they are actually rather unsure of themselves and feel threatened by events or people around them. Believing that you are as good as anyone else and doing things that make you feel good about yourself can make a tremendous difference to your self-esteem and lead to you feeling less anger.

'Anger is often a result of thinking negatively or having a limited number of strategies for dealing with the various situations in which you find yourself,' says Dr Mark McDermott, lecturer and researcher in health psychology at the University of

HOW ANGRY ARE YOU?

Responding to the following statements, as devised in 1989 by Dr McDermott and Professor H.R. Beech, former professor and head of clinical psychology at Manchester University, can help you to identify expressed anger in yourself. How strongly do the following statements apply to you?

1 When things don't go my way I usually end up feeling really irritated with myself.
2 I often find it hard to contain my anger.
3 Sometimes I just get so mad with myself that I feel I could burst with rage.
4 I often get angry with others.
5 If I feel angry I let everyone know in no uncertain terms.
6 I often fly off the handle at others.
7 If someone rejects me it leaves me feeling wounded and bitter.
8 Sometimes I erupt in a blind rage.
9 Sometimes I feel nothing but disrespect and scorn for other people.
10 I often get into fights or arguments with other people.

Score each statement: 1 = untrue of me; 2 = slightly true of me; 3 = moderately true of me; and 4 = very true of me. If you scored lots of 3s and 4s your levels of expressed anger are high and you could find that learning more effective ways of managing your anger is helpful.

East London. Learning to be more flexible in the way you deal with situations can often help. If a particular situation like being stuck in a traffic jam always makes you angry it can help to think of things you could do to help defuse your anger – listening to some calming music or a relaxation tape. If the thing that makes you angry is another person, you could try changing the way you react to the person.

Cognitive behavioural psychologists, who train people in anger management techniques, say that it can help to learn to recognize the stages you go through as you are becoming angry. For example, you might notice your jaw clenching or your stomach tightening. Concentrating on your breathing or practising a relaxation technique at this stage can often nip your anger in the bud. Even if you don't always manage to quell your anger, recognizing that it has a definite pattern can help you feel more in control.

If you are a person who tends to express anger a lot, having an operation to treat your heart disease can be yet another source of anger. Often simply talking to someone – a friend or relative or a professional counsellor or psychologist – can help you to work through your anger. John says: 'I know I was extremely difficult to live with after coming out of hospital. For 18 months after the operation I was kicking the cat – only we don't have a cat. I had great difficulty coming to terms with it. Eventually it was suggested that I see a psychologist at the hospital. She let me offload and pointed me in the direction of an attitude change. Now if the kids are playing up I take half a pace back and ask myself, "Does it really matter?" I'm still quick-fired, a typical Type A, but I do have more control these days about how I react.'

SADNESS AND DEPRESSION

Sadness and crying are also quite common feelings, especially in the period after a heart attack. Depression is more than a feeling of sadness: when you are depressed you feel numb, empty, listless and lacking in energy; things that normally fill you with enthusiasm hold no interest and you are easily irritated. Ken says: 'It was like a blackness. I didn't like being on my own. I felt frightened when I didn't have people around me.'

Other feelings linked with depression are loss of appetite, difficulty sleeping, lack of concentration and suffering aches and pains that make you fear for your health. Some days you may feel better, some worse. This may be linked to how strong you are feeling physically but it is also characteristic of depression.

If you do feel depressed, don't be afraid to express your emotions: you really won't cry for ever even if it feels as though you will at the time, and expressing emotions tends to deprive them of their power. It will also help you to talk to your partner and your friends about how you are feeling. Bear in mind that it is natural to feel sad and grieve when you have lost something. In the case of heart disease these losses include both the real physical damage to your heart and blood vessels and, just as important, your image of yourself as a healthy, active person. Most people become more cheerful again as they regain energy and start to resume their usual activities.

Some people are especially vulnerable to depression. These tend to be people who have experienced previous episodes of depression or who have previously had a lot of loss or hardship in their lives, especially as children. In this case you may need an extra amount of support and help to come to terms with your condition. Sometimes the techniques of cognitive therapy outlined below may help. Sometimes you may need medical help with drugs to help you overcome depression. This is something you should discuss carefully with your doctor.

DEALING WITH EMOTIONS

If you usually refuse to acknowledge your emotions it can be difficult to know exactly how to deal with them. The first step is simply to recognize what you are feeling. Try to be alert to bodily cues such as the lump in your stomach that signals anxiety, the sudden rush of adrenalin that you feel when you are angry, the desire to cry which reveals you are sad.

Once you have identified the emotion you are feeling the next step is to find a way to express it. If you are sad you might choose to have a good old cry or to tell someone you are feeling unhappy. Although a cliché it is still true that a problem shared is often a problem halved. If you feel angry you may decide to remove yourself from the situation, or find a way of venting your feelings. 'Once I had had a few tears I was fine,' remembers John, 'it was a tension release.'

Once you have expressed your feelings the final step is to let them go. You may well find that the strength of your emotions dwindles naturally as time goes on. If it does not you may need to make a more conscious effort to dispense with negative emotions. Some people find it helps to use imagery to visualize getting rid of an emotion. One technique which some counsellors suggest is to imagine packing away your emotion in a drawer. You are allowed to get it out and look at it but afterwards you should put it away again and not dwell on it. If you do this you may well find that it gradually deprives the emotion of its power.

CHANGING THE WAY YOU THINK

Many people who are depressed or anxious view what happens to them in a negative light. Someone who regards life negatively might think, if they have a heart attack: This is the most awful thing that has ever happened. Why is it that terrible things always happen to me? I'll probably die or end up an invalid. I'm never going to be able to cope.

If you have a tendency to think in this way, learning to think more positively can help to lift your mood. You might consciously change your thoughts to the more positive: I've had a heart attack and that's pretty bad. But I am alive; the problem has been sorted out. I've coped before when bad things have happened to me and this heart attack gives me the chance to think about ways of changing my life for the better.

Once you have got the hang of such techniques you can use them to stop your thoughts sliding into a downward spiral whenever you catch yourself thinking negatively. Alternatively, it may help to seek the help of a professional psychotherapist.

Positive thinking techniques such as these are used by psychologists to help people who are suffering from depression in a type of treatment called cognitive therapy. The beauty of this type of therapy is that the techniques can be learnt in just a few sessions, so you do not need to undergo a lengthy course of treatment before you begin to feel better. Research shows that a cognitive therapy can often reverse feelings of depression as successfully as anti-depressant drugs.

WHEN TO SEEK HELP

Most people find their normal mood is restored as they gradually come to terms with the idea of heart disease, but sometimes the uncomfortable feelings don't ease with time. Research suggests a quarter of people who have had a heart attack are experiencing severe psychological problems a year afterwards.

If mood swings, panic attacks or depression last for longer than about six weeks after a diagnosis of heart disease or returning home after a heart attack or surgery, it is important not to feel that you have to struggle on unaided.

If simple reassurance does not help your mood it may help to be referred to a professional psychologist or counsellor who can help you to deal with your feelings; some doctors have such counsellors attached to their practice. Alternatively, your doctor may think it would be helpful to prescribe anti-depressant drugs after you have explained your problems.

SHIFTING RELATIONSHIPS

YOU AND YOUR PARTNER

Research carried out in Germany showed that marriages 'high in intimacy', where the partners find it easy to confide in each other, can protect people who have had a heart attack from anxiety and depression. However, your partner cannot help you if he or she is awash with anxieties of his or her own.

Any crisis, whether it is the discovery that your partner is having an affair, the birth of a new baby or a diagnosis of heart disease, can temporarily unsettle the most stable of relationships. Apart from anything else a diagnosis of heart disease often overturns the balance of a relationship, as Linda points out: 'Here was this man who was always in control and all of a sudden he wasn't in control. It was a difficult time.'

Such role reversal can lead to conflict in a marriage, which if not dealt with can fester and damage the relationship. On the other hand, if each partner feels he or she can safely express his or her fears and weaknesses and the other one can find the strength to deal with them, the relationship can emerge even stronger.

DIFFICULTIES IN CONFIDING

Unfortunately, it is not always easy to confide in each other at such a difficult time, especially if you are someone who is unused to showing emotions, are of a generation that does not discuss emotions freely, or if there are other worries in your relationship.

Although people are much more open nowadays about death and dying, there are still a lot of taboos surrounding any life-threatening illness and it may feel safer to keep your fears and worries to yourself. You may even harbour the superstitious belief that if you admit to being worried about dying it will happen. Exactly how you deal with this will depend very much on the nature of your relationship. If you have always dealt with problems by keeping them to yourself now may not be the time to suddenly start letting them all hang out.

Peter says: 'My wife was diagnosed with breast cancer two years before I had my bypass. She was an enormous support to me even though it must have been very stressful for her. Even so, she never indicated that it was. She was always positive. If she hadn't been I think it would have made it harder for both of us.'

On the other hand both you and your partner may have a real need to air your concerns but be keeping them to yourself to save each other's feelings. If you are usually open and honest with each other keeping your worries bottled up in this way may create a great deal of unnecessary stress, as John and his wife Fiona recall: 'I wanted to talk about it to Fiona but I didn't feel able to,' explains John. 'I was worried about her: she had four young children to look after and now she had a 40-year-old child as well. My reaction was not to tell her stuff. I did it with all the best motives because I wanted to protect her and I felt that by withholding details I could save her from being upset.' Fiona, however, says: 'I felt he was shutting me out. I felt very isolated. I had to pump him for information. We had heated arguments.'

Research has shown that the partners of people who have had a heart attack often have as much need for help and support as the person who had the attack. This is not always forthcoming. You can help your partner by acknowledging their pain and fear. Saying something like, 'I understand how painful it must be for you, I know I would find it hard if it was the other way round,' can open the door to a more honest discussion and an airing of both your fears.

Sad to say, sometimes couples do split up, although this is not likely to happen if your marriage was close to begin with. As Linda, who is also a marriage guidance counsellor, points out: 'It causes you to reassess everything. The person with the heart problem thinks: this is the beginning of the rest of my life and if the marriage hasn't been that wonderful it can be enough to break it up. You have to learn to change your attitude and that can be very difficult.'

LEARNING TO LET GO

Sometimes problems are caused by the person with heart disease using their condition to manipulate other family members. As Professor Bob Lewin points out: 'The person with the heart condition gains power over the family because they hold the unspoken threat, "If you upset me I'm going to die." Family members can become very scared of having an argument in case it provokes a heart attack.'

By the same token, if you are the partner of someone with heart disease you may be tempted to mollycoddle them and never allow them to do anything on their own. The way around both these problems is to try to treat your partner exactly as you would have done before the diagnosis of heart disease, to let go of the illness.

If you are finding it hard to do this, Professor Lewin suggests drawing up a contract whereby the person is allowed to be alone or do whatever it is that the partner is afraid of 'for a negotiated and mutually agreed period of time'. An example might be going for a walk unaccompanied. The initial period may need to be quite short, say a ten-minute walk once a day. It is essential that the patient sticks to the contract and does not take the opportunity to slip away for a longer period. After a week of such walks a new and longer period can be negotiated. Treated in this way the period of separation can usually be extended systematically and the partner's anxiety will gradually subside.'

GETTING SUPPORT

Supportive though your partner, friends and family may be, some of your nearest and dearest may appear insensitive to your needs. This may simply be because of their own desire to put what has happened to you behind them and re-establish a sense of normality. A gentle reminder that you still need help and support may be all that is needed to get a more sensitive response.

If you live alone, friends and relatives are likely to be your main source of support. You will probably find that many friends are more than willing to lend a listening ear or help you in some practical ways, but some will not want to appear intrusive or think that you want to forget about your disease. If people aren't forthcoming, don't be afraid to make it clear that you welcome their support and encouragement.

It can sometimes be helpful to talk to someone outside the family, such as a cardiac nurse, a specially trained counsellor or health visitor, as Carolyn found out: 'I wanted people to listen but I felt some of my friends and family didn't understand because they don't know what it was like. Some were more receptive than others. Other people think you're all right now, but you do need a sympathetic ear. It was good to have someone outside the family, someone who was impersonal. I felt she really did understand. She was very gentle and that was just what I needed.'

John says: 'I used to talk to Ali (the cardiac counsellor). I felt it was safer to talk to someone else. Fiona, with the best will in the world, didn't know what the answers were.'

Fiona for her part found it helpful to write things down after John's second bypass: 'I didn't want to offload my worries on to the kids, even though they were older. I thought I couldn't start blubbing in front of them but I did need someone to talk to. John and I would always sit down and start bantering with each other after the kids have gone to bed. Now he was in hospital there was no one to do that with. I didn't want to start ringing friends and relatives at that time of night, so I used that time to keep a diary. For me it served two purposes. The first was to ease my anxiety. The second was to see his progress. Although it didn't feel progress at the time – it felt very slow – it was almost like a map of how it was going.'

FRIENDS YOU COULD DO WITHOUT

One of the less appealing human traits is a tendency to revel in the misfortunes of others. Some people you know or meet will positively delight in regaling you in horrific detail with tales of their own heart attacks or operations or those of people they know. 'Before my bypass,' recalls Sylvia, 'some people frightened me by telling me how painful it would be. In my opinion it is not as terrible as people make out. It is painful but it's bearable pain.'

There are various ways to combat the horror stories. Avoidance is one tactic, for example by putting off meetings to a later date or hiding behind the answerphone. Arming yourself with accurate facts so you can counter negative information is another. It may be worth taking the time to explain the true facts about heart disease to people who are close to you, who may simply not be *au fait* with all the advances that have taken place over the past few years. On the other hand, especially if the person concerned is not especially important to you, you may decide that you do not really want him or her in your life at all and choose to let your acquaintanceship lapse altogether.

SUPPORT GROUPS

One way both people with heart disease and their partners can share some of the burden is to join a support group. People who have had a heart problem often feel no one quite understands as well as someone who has been through it too. 'After Len had seen his cardiologist we went on holiday to Tenerife,' Linda explains. 'While we were sitting on the beach one day a gentleman with a scar down his chest just like Len's came up and said, "I see you are in the club." They had never seen each other before but they sat there for at least two hours talking together like long-lost friends, comparing notes. They seemed to derive such comfort and strength from each other, that I realized what the importance of self-help groups could be.'

In many areas there are now local heart support groups, or chapters as they are called in the US. Some of these are based at hospitals, others are affiliated to heart charities. The British Heart Foundation has almost 200 affiliated support groups and in the USA there are similar groups operating under the auspices of Mended Hearts, affiliated to the AHA.

'The aim is to provide up-to-date information and to encourage people to make and maintain long-term lifestyle changes,' explains Jackie Sutcliffe, a British Heart Foundation support group adviser in Yorkshire. 'Some groups are exercise-based, others organize walks, dances and other social events.' Many groups have their own telephone lines which you can call for extra help and support if you need to.

Jackie Sutcliffe says that partners often benefit as much or even more than the person with heart disease. 'The patient receives lots of help and advice, while the wife or husband is often left to deal with it on their own. Sharing feelings with other people who have been through the same experience that you have been through and understand your emotions can be tremendously reassuring.'

Support groups are not for everyone. Some people simply don't like joining groups and prefer to come to terms with their illness in their own way and their own time. Others may come to feel that the group does not meet their particular needs – if you are a woman you may feel the group is biased towards men, for example. You may also feel nervous about attending on your own. This is not necessary, because while many support groups do encourage partners to attend it is not a condition of joining. If you do pluck up the courage to go along you will almost certainly find people friendly and welcoming. It also has to be said that some heart support groups themselves are downbeat: Jim describes one he went to as 'full of people sitting around moping and moaning'.

If you are unsure about joining it may be a good idea to go along for a couple of sessions and try to establish the tone of the group. If you feel a particular group is not for you there is no need to feel guilty if you choose not to continue to attend. On the other hand, you could try to change it from within by getting involved in organizing activities.

Many people find that after they have recovered from a heart attack, surgery or whatever they eventually want to put the experience behind them. Norma Jackson, secretary of the UK's Zipper Club, for people who have had bypass surgery says: 'People join the group after having heart surgery because they feel quite vulnerable but most give up after about a year. I consider that a sign of success.'

WHAT DO WE TELL THE CHILDREN?

A family is a unit and what happens to one of its members can send ripples through to all the others no matter how young.

John says: 'I remember hearing about a teenage boy whose father went into hosptital for a heart operation. The child really started rebelling and ended up seeing a counsellor. It emerged that the child had been left out of the picture completely; it was mother and father who coped with everything and the child was angry at his father for having a heart problem. His way of reacting was to play up. That made such an impact on me; I was determined we would be open with our children.'

How much you decide to tell your children will depend very much on what your condition is and their ages. Very young children may not need to be told very much if you simply have angina which is being treated. However, if you have been rushed to hospital with a heart attack or been taken in for surgery or another procedure, even young children will need to know in simple terms what has happened.

Fiona says: 'In a way it was easier that our children were so young because there was only a limited amount they could understand. We told them that Dad had to go for an operation and would be in hospital for a while. I took them to visit him a couple of days later and later on he showed them his scar. That seemed a very natural thing to do. Natalie, who was one, didn't know much and Christopher, who was three, didn't really react. I remember he made John a card with all the nurses on it. But

Christine, who was then seven, was very shocked by the scar. We went through what had happened but there is only so much you can tell. There is no point in giving them a load of information that goes over their heads.'

Older children and teenagers can understand more and may benefit from a more detailed explanation. However, they may feel irritated by what they perceive as demands to return to the family fold at a time when they are struggling with their own task of establishing a separate identity. Fiona says: 'By the time John had his second bypass five years later they were all much older, but by then we'd started the Cardiac Club, so they'd seen cardiac patients and it was less of an event. We still had a few tears on the day, mind you.'

Older children may still need the opportunity to air their fears and worries, and if they find it difficult to talk to you it may help if they can confide in an understanding grandparent, teacher, school counsellor or adult friend.

SEX MATTERS

One of the biggest causes of anxiety after a diagnosis of heart disease is often sex. Sex can be many things: relief, fun, a way of feeling close to your partner, a way of communicating, a physical expression of your love and affection for each other or, if you are just embarking on a new relationship, a way of moving the relationship on to a more intimate footing.

Although sexual problems can sometimes be a result of the drugs prescribed, by far the greatest problem is that having heart disease can affect your sense of self-worth and this in turn has a knock-on effect on the desire to make love. 'Both the person with heart disease and their partner have to come to terms with the change from seeing themselves as an active, healthy person who could do what they liked to someone who may have limitations on their activities,' explains John Lenkiewicz, director of the UK's Institute of Sexuality and Human Relations.

SEX AFTER A HEART ATTACK

'In particular, people often worry about resuming sex after a heart attack because they fear that sex will induce another attack,' says John Lenkiewicz. The fact is there is only a very minute risk (around one in a million) of sex triggering a heart attack – although there is some evidence that having sex with someone who isn't your regular partner may be more risky. Even in this situation it is important to keep a sense of perspective and to bear in mind that any increased risk is very, very small. Encouragingly, research shows that those who are sexually active have a lower risk of having another attack, which makes sense when you consider that, apart from anything else, sex is a form of exercise.

SEX AFTER SURGERY

After surgery worries may be focused on the scar and the fear of damaging it in some way. Fiona says: 'It was difficult to get back to a normal sex life at first. I felt frightened. After the operation John went to rehab so he knew what he could do, but all I could see was the scar. I thought, Oh my God, if I put pressure on his breast bone he'll collapse, or if I get him too excited his heart will go into overload. John made the first approach and my answer was, "You'll hurt yourself." He just said, "Don't be stupid." It's fear of the unknown, really. Once we got going again and I knew what he could and couldn't do it was fine, but it was a gradual process. Interestingly enough, he still has this sensitivity across the chest where nerve endings were severed.'

Strangely, having surgery can actually give your sex life a new lease of life,' says Linda. 'Before the surgery it may have diminished because the person was feeling rotten. They may have put this down to the fact that they are getting older. The first time you think, Gosh, is he going to die? but once you get over that it's all right.'

'The best way to diffuse such anxieties to be honest with each other,' advises John Lenkiewicz. Admitting to the way you are feeling opens the way for a free and open discussion that can allay fears you have and help you to feel closer. 'One of the best ways of building up your self-esteem,' he advises, 'is to "greet life again". This means that, having had the experience and lived through it, you start working or doing things you enjoy and feeling that life is agreable once more. Forcing yourself to live as if you feel good about yourself in the end helps you to feel better.'

HEART MEDICATION AND SEX

It has to be admitted that some of the medications used to treat heart disease can, in a small number of men, affect the ability to have an erection. The main culprits are beta-blockers and diuretics. Doctors sometimes keep quiet about this in the belief that people taking the drugs will anticipate problems and therefore create them. It is certainly true that 'performance anxiety' can be the real reason behind the inability to achieve an erection, but it is as well to be aware of potential side effects so that you do not blame yourself if you do experience difficulties.

Relax and try not to anticipate problems. If you do suspect that a drug you are taking is causing erectile difficulties it is worth having a word with your doctor. There is a wide variety of heart drugs available nowadays and it is often possible to change you on to one that doesn't affect your ability to have an erection.

LET'S GET PHYSICAL

During sex breathing becomes more rapid, the heart rate rises and blood pressure increases slightly. Physically, for the heart, sex is about the equivalent of walking briskly up a couple of flights of stairs. This has led experts to recommend that, provided you can manage 20 steps without experiencing chest pain and other symptoms, it should be safe to have sex.

There are no set rules about when you should start having sex again, although some doctors recommend waiting until the second week after you come out of hospital if you have had surgery or a heart attack. Using your GTN spray to pre-empt angina, if necessary, can help make life easier.

By and large it is best to be guided by your body and your desire. Try not to expect too much too soon and view any occasional setbacks or disappointments as just that, 'occasional'. Relax and laugh them off. Don't let them become huge obstacles. When you feel ready to resume your sex life, take it slowly and gradually. In the meantime express your love and affection for each other in different ways with hugs, caresses, kisses, stroking and holding hands. The following tips may be helpful:

- Although many people in the UK like to keep their bedrooms cooler than the rest of the house, if you have heart disease it's a good idea to keep your bedroom at a warm, comfortable temperature. Going from a warm environment to a cool one can spark off a bout of angina, which can be a sure-fire dampener to desire.

- For the same reason you may like to warm the sheets with an electric blanket so you don't have to get into a cold bed.

- There are no positions which are recommended or inadvisable, although immediately after surgery it may be preferable to choose positions in which the person who has had surgery is on top, to avoid putting pressure on the chest.

- It is best to avoid having sex within a couple of hours of eating a heavy meal, and to steer clear of alcohol for a few hours before going to bed too, for the traditional reason that it 'increases the desire but takes away the performance'.

- Long, exhausting marathon sex sessions are best avoided. Make your lovemaking langorous and leisurely and be prepared to take an occasional break. Tell the doctor if you experience symptoms such as severe fatigue, breathlessness or angina.

NEW PARTNERS

If you are single, separated, widowed or divorced you may worry about how to cope if you meet a potential partner. The early stages of a new relationship are often very intense and you may worry about telling your new partner about your heart condition and how it will affect your sex life. You may be afraid that your new partner will reject you. As in other situations, honesty is by far the best policy and will help allay any anxiety. As far as actual lovemaking is concerned the same guidelines apply as for people with a regular partner.

CHAPTER 9

HEART DISEASE AND WOMEN

'My first heart attack wasn't recognized at all. Not until I was rushed to hospital with what they thought was typhoid fever and it was actually a massive heart attack. They said I was too young.'

BRITISH HEART FOUNDATION LEAFLET, WOMEN AND HEART DISEASE

If YOU WERE ASKED TO SAY what sort of person was most likely to develop heart disease you would almost certainly describe a middle-aged, overweight man in a stressful job. As so often with stereotypes not is this only a partial picture but it is one that may be harmful. It is true that more men have heart attacks than women and also that men have them earlier in life, but one in nine women between 45 and 64 have heart disease and from the age of 65 onwards a woman's risk of developing heart disease catches up with a man's.

Statistics can present a confused and often distorted picture. To read that, according to American Heart Association figures, 44 per cent of women die within a year of a heart attack compared to 27 per cent of men, is worrying but requires a little thought: since women are, statistically, older when they develop heart disease, they are also less likely to survive because of their *age*, not solely their *gender*. There is also evidence that women may delay going to the doctor, playing down early symptoms and putting their family's health before their own and not finding time to attend rehabilitation programmes. However, in the UK it is estimated that around 67,000 women die of a heart attack each year. What is more, a quarter of deaths are in women under 45.

THE CHALLENGE FOR WOMEN

That's the bad news. The good news is that research shows that women with angina are less likely to have furring and narrowing of the arteries than men (the symptoms are often caused by spasm of the arteries – a condition known as Syndrome X). At the same time women are more likely to live longer than men once angina has developed.

Another encouraging fact, according to a 1997 article in the *Lancet* called 'Women's Hearts are Hard to Break', is that women's risk of dying from coronary heart disease by the age of 65 is still only one in 70. Even more encouragingly, a report in 1997 in the *British Medical Journal* suggests that a woman's increased risk of dying after a heart attack is limited to the first 30 days after an attack.

So that puts the risks in perspective. On the other hand, if you have developed heart disease the figures do underline how important it is to do everything you can to reduce your risk factors. They also suggest that you may need to be especially assertive to get the best possible care from the medical profession. As consultant cardiologist Graham Jackson puts it in an article in the *British Medical Journal*: 'Women are different – but not that different. Although women with coronary artery disease may be more difficult to diagnose and manage than men it is a challenge that we *and they* [my italics] must rise to.'

COMBATTING RISK FACTORS

Women share many of the same risk factors for heart disease as men such as family history, age, blood pressure, smoking and cholesterol levels. However, research suggests that because of their biology some of these factors affect women slightly differently. Gill says: 'My cholesterol levels are OK but of course I was a smoker. My older brother had a heart attack too, so possibly there is a family connection. In fact, although I did not know it before my mother told me, my grandmother died of heart attack.'

Reducing your risk factors, watching what you eat and exercising are just as important for women as they are for men. Research shows that although women tend to live longer on the whole than men, in later life they may be more unhealthy than men. As well as heart disease women are at risk of osteoporosis (brittle bone disease), arthritis and breast and other cancers. One of the bonuses of following a healthy lifestyle is that the same factors of exercise and a healthy diet that protect against heart disease also have a protective effect against these other diseases.

HORMONAL CONNECTIONS

The female sex hormone, oestrogen, is thought to be one of the most important factors in the development of heart disease in women. Before the menopause oestrogen seems to have a protective effect on the arteries. This may be because it acts as an anti-oxidant, helping to mop up free radicals, the harmful molecules that are believed to be involved in the development of atherosclerosis.

Oestrogen may not be the only significant factor, however. Some scientists now think that there may be something else that protects pre-menopausal women against heart disease. An American Heart Association study suggest that **prostaglandins**, hormone-like substances secreted by the uterus, may also have a protective effect against heart disease. One of the jobs of some prostaglandins is to control the smooth muscle activity of the blood vessels (they are involved in stimulating contractions in labour, for instance); other prostaglandins are involved in blood clotting. Both these factors are, of course, of relevance in heart disease. Although the research is only at an early stage it could prove very exciting.

The Pill

As so often with issues concerning the Pill, the relationship between the Pill and heart disease is not entirely clear, and evidence is often conflicting and contradictory.

Taking the Pill affects levels of hormones and other substances, such as blood fats, in the body. Some types of Pill (notably the high-dose combined variety) raise blood pressure in some women.

Research has also linked taking the Pill with an increased risk of having both a stroke and developing a blood clot in the veins (deep venous thrombosis). The risks are even higher if you smoke. Taking the Pill, though, does not seem to raise the risk of atherosclerosis and some studies suggest that it may even help protect against this factor in heart disease.

There is also concern about the use of the Pill and breast cancer (although the latest British studies suggest that the risk dwindles after you stop taking the Pill and is returned to normal after ten years). When making decisions about taking the Pill, therefore, you need to take into account both your own medical and family medical history and your need for birth control.

PREGNANCY

Pregnancy affects all the body's functions. During pregnancy the heart has to work harder as the body's blood volume increases by half to supply the needs of the baby. There is also a higher risk of blood clotting and blood pressure may rise in the final few weeks of pregnancy. The most extreme form of this rise in blood pressure is the 'pregnancy disease', pre-eclampsia.

The body adapts to pregnancy and these factors do not make any significant difference to women without heart disease. However, if you already have angina or other symptoms of heart disease you will need expert advice and monitoring. Belinda Linden, nurse adviser at the British Heart Foundation, writing in the BHF's *Newsbeat*, says: 'Many women can manage quite well if there are few or no symptoms before pregnancy.'

Your pregnancy and postnatal care will be shared between your obstetrician and cardiologist. Certain drugs may need to be changed during pregnancy to avoid harming the unborn baby.

AGE AND THE MENOPAUSE

Women, like men, are more at risk of heart disease as they get older. With age, the levels of both total cholesterol and 'bad' LDL cholesterol rise, and it is difficult to tease out the effects of the menopause from the effects of simply getting older.

A recent study carried out in Norway of 20,000 women over a 29-year period found that women who experienced an early menopause (before the age of 44) were over twice as likely to develop a fatal heart condition as those who had their menopause after the age of 53. This seems to add weight to the theory that before the menopause oestrogen has a significant protective effect against furred arteries.

Hormone replacement therapy (HRT)

The question of whether to take hormone replacement therapy, HRT (ERT in the US), is complicated for all women. Some studies show that the risk of heart disease is almost halved if you take HRT; others suggest that the risk of thrombosis and stroke are increased.

The ingredient in HRT which is most beneficial for women's hearts is oestrogen. The type of HRT known as 'unopposed' contains oestrogen only, but women who haven't had a hysterectomy are prescribed a type of HRT called 'opposed', which contains progestogens, synthetic forms of another female sex hormone, progesterone. This protects the uterus against cancer of the womb lining – a risk with unopposed HRT – but it is not yet entirely clear what the effects of progestogens are on the heart.

The benefits of taking HRT as a protection against heart disease also have to be weighed against the risk of developing breast cancer, which rises as women get older. Studies have shown that taking HRT over time does boost the risk of breast cancer. Of course, this has to be balanced against its beneficial effects on the heart, especially when you consider the fact that heart disease kills more women than breast cancer.

If you are thinking about taking HRT, talk it over thoroughly with your family doctor or a physician who specializes in the menopause. You will need to think very carefully about the risks and benefits in the light of your own personal medical history and risk factors. You might want to take some of the following into account:

- If you are at high risk of developing heart disease due to high cholesterol, family history or other factors it is well worth considering HRT.
- If you are at a fairly low risk of heart disease you may be less likely to need HRT but might still benefit from it for relief of menopausal symptoms such as hot flushes or preventing osteoporosis (brittle bone disease) and later heart disease.
- If you have a personal or family history of uterine or breast cancer you may want to avoid HRT.

If you already have heart disease, diabetes, high blood pressure or have had a stroke, doctors say that there is no reason to avoid HRT but you will need to discuss all the risks and benefits in your particular case with your doctor.

OBTAINING A DIAGNOSIS

Gill recalls the difficulty she experienced in getting a diagnosis: 'I first became aware that there was something wrong when I began to slow down at work. My job was quite high-powered and I noticed that when I was out with my assistant, who is not that much younger than me, I couldn't keep up. Occasionally I had dizzy spells. I half-suspected that there was something wrong with my heart and saw the doctor. She did a resting ECG which showed nothing.'

After Gill had seen her family doctor she continued to feel unwell and decided to see a consultant cardiologist through her firm's private insurance scheme: 'He sent me for a stress test. During it I felt dizzy, peculiar and breathless, but again nothing showed up. The consultant said, "All the tests show nothing but I'm not happy. If you come in tomorrow we'll do an angiogram." I realized something was probably wrong because he kept saying, "Let me see that bit again."'

Eventually the consultant told Gill there was something he couldn't quite see and that he wanted to do a thallium test, in which a radioactive substance is injected into the bloodstream and which can show areas where the heart is blocked or damaged. The scan revealed that the aorta, the large artery that receives blood from the left ventricle and circulates it to the rest of the body, was blocked. The tests that Gill underwent are explained in Chapter 2.

Gill subsequently had heart bypass surgery. She feels that it is important to trust your instincts if you are experiencing symptoms that might indicate heart disease.

It is a fact that women may find it more difficult to get a diagnosis than men and Gill's experience is echoed in scientific research. There may be several reasons for this. For a start, the doctor may be less likely to be looking for heart disease if you are a woman, especially if you have not yet gone through the menopause. Research shows that women, especially younger women, are less likely than men to be investigated for heart disease – and of course if you are not investigated it is impossible to reach a diagnosis.

Secondly, women tend to experience more atypical symptoms than men. As we have already seen, while men are more likely to have a heart attack as their first symptom, women are more likely to complain of angina. However, classic angina symptoms are less common in women too. If you are a woman you should never ignore chest pains that occur as a result of activity or put them down to indigestion. You should also look carefully at the atypical symptoms listed in Chapter 1.

Finally, some diagnostic tests seem to be less useful in women with heart disease. In women under 65, for example, exercise testing seems to throw up more false-positive results (over 65 it is as useful for women as for men). Other tests such as a thallium scan or echocardiography may be less clear-cut, too, because breast tissue may obscure the heart.

What this means is that as a woman you may have to be prepared to be especially assertive and persistent if you are worried about any symptoms.

GETTING TREATMENT

There is evidence to suggest that women with heart disease receive less intensive drug treatment than men. For instance, one study showed that women were less likely to receive clotbusting drugs during a heart attack. Another study found that beta-blockers were given less often to women than to men when they left hospital after a heart attack. Drugs may also affect women differently – ACE inhibitors, for example, have sometimes been shown to cause a cough more often in women than in men.

WOMEN AND HEART SURGERY

Research also suggests that women are not referred for surgery as often as men and that women who have surgery are more severely ill. One explanation for this could be that, statistically, women with heart disease are older and therefore may have other physical illnesses that might prolong their recovery period, so doctors may be more reluctant to advise surgery. The latest research, however, shows that women do just as well – and in some cases even better – both physically and in reports of improved quality of life and vitality. What these findings underline is the importance for women with heart disease to make sure that they have explored all the options for treatment with their doctor.

Much of what has been written about recovering from surgery in Chapter 5 applies to women as well as men. Women may find it particularly uncomfortable to wear a bra after surgery and because women's clothes tend to expose their bodies more than men's there may be one or two extra issues to consider. Gill recalls the shock at the state of her legs, which were cut open to remove a suitable vein for her bypass. 'Now they swell up and I can't stand for long. It is very annoying as I had nice legs and used to like wearing mini skirts. Now I wear trousers most of time and very rarely wear a dress. I can't wear low-cut things either because of the scar on my chest.'

AFTER A HEART ATTACK

As already mentioned, research shows that women do less well than men in the 30 days after a heart attack. It is therefore especially important to pace yourself and not to go back to running the household straight away when you come out of hospital after a heart attack. Allow yourself time, too, for attending rehabilitation sessions and some gentle exercise. It is also important to be aware of the warning signs of another heart attack outlined in Chapter 1.

A UK study carried out at Liverpool University in 1997 looking at emotional responses after a heart attack found that women experienced even more emotional difficulties than men after a heart attack and reported a significantly poorer emotional quality of life. 'Women tend to be more emotional in their reaction to having a heart attack and often need more support than men,' observes BHF nurse Karen Caffrey. 'Men have often been conditioned to think that it is not manly to express feelings openly and bottle them up; women tend to be more open in expressing their emotions.' This is no bad thing, as expressing your emotions can enable you to get the help and support you need.

REHABILITATION

It has been found that women are less likely to attend the supervised rehabilitation programmes run by many hospitals. This may be because they feel self-conscious that there are fewer women than men in the group, or because they feel the information and exercise is geared more towards men. The British Heart Foundation observes in their leaflet, *Women and Heart Disease*: 'A reluctance to start becoming more active is possibly one of the main reasons women do not do so well as men when they have heart disease.'

For this reason it is well worth trying to overcome your feelings of discomfort and sticking at a rehabilitation programme if you have the chance to join one. Alternatively, try to follow the other tips on becoming more active given in Chapter 5.

OBTAINING PRACTICAL HELP AND SUPPORT

'Returning home is also sometimes more difficult for women than men because men, especially those of the older generation, tend to get looked after by their wives while women are expected to go back and start doing the housework and look after the family again straight away,' points out Karen Caffrey. It is important to allow yourself enough time to recover properly. Be guided by your body and energy levels and don't push yourself to do too much, especially if you also have a job outside the home. Keep housework to the bare minimum and be prepared to let standards drop for a while. Encourage your partner, if you have one, to help with the cooking and cleaning or, if you can afford it, consider paying for a home help. Take up any offers of help from family and friends.

If talking to friends and relatives is not enough you may benefit from professional counselling. Ask your doctor if you can be referred. Some doctors now offer counselling in their surgeries.

CHAPTER 10

COMPLEMENTARY THERAPIES

'You need to work at a deeper level. So many people in our culture are isolated, lonely and unhappy. If we don't address that underlying pain, telling patients they will live longer is not always a powerful motivator.'

DR DEAN ORNISH, REPORTED IN *PHYSICIAN AND SPORTSMEDICINE*, 1994

SOONER OR LATER MANY PEOPLE WITH A CHRONIC ILLNESS such as heart disease think about trying complementary therapies. Conventional medicine is very good at saving lives in an acute situation such as a heart attack but for ongoing problems the complementary route may seem to offer a better prospect of feeling in control. And this, as we have already seen, is an important step on the road to recovery. In practice, only a small percentage of people with heart disease pursue this route, but this chapter looks at why you might decide to seek complementary treatment, how to choose a therapy that is suitable and details of some of the complementary therapies that are said to be especially helpful for heart disease.

WHY GO COMPLEMENTARY?

Social psychologists Adrian Furnham and Bruce Kirkcaldy confirm that the opportunity to take a more active part in treatment is one the most potent reasons people are attracted towards complementary therapies. With their emphasis on treating the whole person, such therapies may seem to offer a more individual and personal approach.

Many of us, according to Furnham and Kirkcaldy, feel frustrated by what we see as the failure of orthodox medicine and prefer the idea of therapies that offer a more natural, gentle and relaxing way of treating illness. Worries about the adverse effects of orthodox drugs or surgery are often another factor.

Greta, for example, explains her motives for seeking chelation therapy (see below): 'I developed angina when I was 40 and when I was 41 was offered a bypass. It worked well for a time but by the time I was 46 my symptoms had become so bad again I was told I needed another one. I thought, Hang on, I'm only a young woman, this doesn't seem to be the answer. So I decided to give chelation a whirl. I realize that my problem is never likely to go away altogether but it has made life so much more tolerable. I am able to live a more reasonable lifestyle. It has cost a lot of money but you can't put a price on your health, can you?'

Finally, according to Furnham and Kirkaldy people often seek out non-orthodox treatments because they are dissatisfied with the way their doctors communicate and feel that an alternative or complementary practitioner will give them more time and listen more sympathetically.

MAKING A POSITIVE CHOICE

Choosing to use complementary therapies, of course, is not usually an either/or option. Most people who use such treatments do so alongside medical treatment and you may even find that your doctor has one or more complementary therapists, such as a homeopath, acupuncturist and so on working at the surgery.

Turning to complementary therapies as a way of solving problems with your orthodox doctor is rarely a good reason to go complementary. As someone with a chronic illness you are bound to have some long-term contact with your doctor. So, unless you have decided to go the whole hog and reject orthodox medicine altogether, it is worth making an effort to get your relationship on a reasonable footing.

If communication between you and your orthodox doctor leaves something to be desired, try to think of ways in which you can improve it, for example by arranging an extra-long appointment to find out exactly what you want to know about your condition. If you and your doctor really cannot get on it may be worth changing your doctor.

Similarly, if you are worried about the side effects of any drugs you have been prescribed it is worth trying to sort this out directly with your doctor. You should never just suddenly stop taking drugs prescribed for heart disease as it may be dangerous.

As for the claim that complementary therapies are natural

and therefore gentle, it is worth making the point that some alternative medicines, such as herbs, have just as powerful effects as synthetic drugs. They should be prescribed and used with extreme care. For this reason it is always better to seek the help of a qualified practitioner rather than trying to treat yourself.

Finally, it has to be said some alternative practitioners can be just as, or even more, dogmatic in their approach as the most intractable orthodox cardiologist.

None of this is intended to dissuade you from seeking out complementary help. Rather, it is intended to help ensure that you approach such therapies with the same informed eye you would (hopefully) apply to any form of treatment.

THE CONVENTIONAL MEDICAL VIEW

Some complementary therapies, such as relaxation techniques, yoga and others, are now found on many rehabilitation programmes and recommended by conventional doctors. If you do decide to go complementary you may be pleasantly surprised by your doctor's response, as Barbara Rowlands, author of *The Which? Guide to Complementary Medicine*, points out: 'Some doctors are still opposed to complementary treatments but they tend to be the older ones. Four out of ten doctors now offer complementary therapies, so they are not all against them and so long as you are taking the correct drugs most would be quite happy to endorse complementary therapy and some may even offer it under the NHS.'

Your doctor, not surprisingly, will be considerably less happy if you decide to reject conventional treatment altogether. However, this may be an option you wish to pursue if conventional treatment has failed, you have reached the point where the doctor has told you that no further treatment can be offered, or if you are feeling so thoroughly disillusioned with mainstream medicine that you feel you want to try something else.

Greta says: 'My doctor has been very encouraging and interested and is convinced that chelation therapy has worked for me. The health authority say it is all in the mind and will not fund my treatment. My cardiologist was not keen, but I told him because I wanted to make sure he would continue to treat me. Afterwards he could see how much I had improved but he said the only way to prove it was to go for another angiogram and I was not prepared to do that. He then took the attitude, "Well, people develop collaterals". He is not convinced.'

Even if you do expect to meet opposition it is still worth telling your doctor you are having complementary treatment. Feeling unsupported by your medical advisers can in itself be a source of stress. Certainly if you are planning to take anything pharmacologically active, such as herbs or supplements, your doctor should know.

SELECTING A THERAPY

There is a huge number of complementary therapies available. If you like the idea of trying one it can be quite hard to decide which one to choose. Buying a book and reading about what is available will enable you to see what is on offer. When it comes to choosing one, Barbara Rowlands offers the following advice: 'I think it is terribly important that complementary therapy is not used for potentially fatal diseases. If you have got a serious heart problem obviously you should go to your doctor first of all. The majority of complementary therapists who are well trained and belong to a reputable organization would treat a heart patient with great care. However, I would advise any heart patient to be careful and go for the gentler complementary therapies and avoid anything that is harsh or invasive. Patients could try hatha yoga or t'ai chi, for example, rather than iyengar yoga, which would be too rough. Massage is wonderful for relaxation, but again I would advise going for a soft sort such as Swedish massage, aromatherapy or reflexology rather than something like rolfing.'

Barbara Rowlands also warns people with heart disease against any therapy which involves fasting. 'People are sometimes told to fast to get rid of toxins from the body. However, most people don't have toxins and fasting puts an enormous strain on the body which could be harmful for anyone with a heart condition.'

CHOOSING A PRACTITIONER

It is often pointed out that many complementary practitioners do not have the detailed medical knowledge doctors have. Nor are all registered with a regulatory body as doctors have to be. This may not matter: the healing skills of therapists of both orthodox and complementary persuasion often owe as much to intangibles such as the relationship between healer and healed as they do to pills and potions. There are good and bad doctors just as there are good and bad complementary practitioners.

If you do decide to seek complementary treatment bear in mind that there is rather more of an onus on you to make sure that you choose someone who is reliable. It makes sense to steer clear of anyone who offers you a miracle cure, especially if they are demanding large sums of money for it. Some doctors may be willing to recommend a practitioner, and in the UK it is sensible to check with the Institute of Complementary Medicine, which keeps a register of accredited practitioners (see Useful Addresses). It can be helpful to listen to other people's experiences, but bear in mind that yours will not necessarily be the same.

THE LIFESTYLE HEART TRIAL

Cardiologists have always maintained that, although much can be done to slow the progression of atherosclerosis with drugs and surgery and by tackling risk factors, nothing can actually stop it, still less reverse it. In the past few years, however, a few doctors have begun to modify their views slightly. The change of heart has partly come about in the light of the evidence that medical treatments such as cholesterol-lowering drugs can reverse atherosclerosis, but some experts have gone one step further than this and argue that the same effects can be achieved solely by making changes in lifestyle.

Perhaps the most surprising – and encouraging – thing about this is that the trial that started it all off was conducted not by a 'cranky' alternative therapist but by the assistant clinical professor of medicine at the University of California, Dr Dean Ornish. Dr Ornish's report, *Can Lifestyle Changes Reverse Coronary Heart Disease?*, which was published in the *Lancet* in July 1990, caused an immediate storm in the world of cardiology.

The study followed a group of 48 people with established coronary artery disease which had been confirmed by angiography. Of the group, 28 were put on a rigorous low-fat vegetarian diet containing just 10 per cent fat. They were also instructed to take a minimum three hours per week of moderate exercise and to follow a stress management programme consisting of an hour's daily stretching exercises, breathing techniques, meditation, progressive relaxation and imagery designed,

THE LIFESTYLE DIET

- **Allowed in unlimited quantities**
  Fruits   Vegetables   Grains   Pulses and soya bean products

- **Forbidden**
  Animal products (apart from egg white and one cup per day
  of non-fat milk or yoghurt)
  Caffeine
  Salt (for those with high blood pressure)

- **Allowed in limited quantities**
  Two units of alcohol per day

- **Energy balance**
  Fat: 10 per cent of calories
  Protein: 15–20 per cent of calories
  Complex carbohydrates: 70–75 per cent of calories
  Cholesterol: 5mg a day or less

according to the *Lancet*, 'to increase relaxation, concentration and awareness'. The remaining 20, acting as a control group, were told to adhere to the standard advice given to heart patients, such as cutting fat to 30 per cent, taking moderate exercise and so on.

The group started the programme with a week-long stay in a hotel where they were instructed in the changes they were required to make. Subsequently they attended regular group support meetings twice weekly.

Strikingly, people on the programme experienced an improvement in their angina after just a few days. A year later they had 91 per cent fewer angina attacks, attacks lasted for a shorter time and were less severe. Their levels of blood fats were similar to those seen with cholesterol-lowering drugs. Even more astonishingly, atherosclerosis had actually begun to reverse in 18 of the 22 people (six dropped out). By contrast, those in the control group who followed more conventional advice suffered more frequent and severe attacks of angina and experienced a worsening of their atherosclerosis.

Ornish's research is tremendously exciting because it opens up the possibility of treating heart disease naturally without the need for drugs or surgery. Despite this, conventional cardiologists have not by and large greeted it with enthusiasm. Some point out that the group was only small and and that it would not be possible or practical to treat large groups of people in this way. They also argue that the programme demands considerably more dedication than could be expected of the average heart patient. The diet – strictly vegetarian with a minimum of dairy products, and one-third the fat usually recommended – takes a lot of getting used to, while the stress management programme of at least an hour a day also demands a very high level of commitment. The group also had a tremendous amount of support and encouragement to stick at the programme and critics often maintain that without this high level of back-up – impractical with large groups or on an impoverished health service – it would be more difficult for people to maintain the necessary changes.

THE SPIRITUAL DIMENSION

Dr Ornish himself argues that it is often easier for people to make really sweeping changes than more moderate ones. Where he really parts company with many of his more conventionally minded colleagues is in his belief that heart disease is linked to the lack of spirituality found in modern Western societies.

Of course, it is less easy to prove such a belief than it is to show that a certain drug or even lifestyle change works. What research does show is that people with heart disease who are depressed seem to have a poorer long-term outlook than those who think more positively. Research also suggests that having a supportive partner and strong relationships seems to make a big difference to how well people do. While such research does not explain how spiritual and emotional factors might be important in heart disease it certainly lends weight to Dr Ornish's theory.

MEDITATION MATTERS

One feature of Dr Ornish's programme which has attracted a lot of research in its own right is meditation, in particular **Transcendental Meditation** or TM, introduced to the West by the Maharishi Mahesh Yogi in the 1960s.

Some 500 studies have been published on TM over the past 25 years. These suggest that the technique is effective in lowering blood pressure and cholesterol, improving angina, increasing resistance to stress and reducing other risk factors for heart disease such as smoking, obesity and depression. One US study showed that over five years people who meditated were 87 per cent less likely to go into hospital with heart disease.

Critics tend to point out that many of these research studies were carried out by scientists within the Maharishi Foundation and published in journals which are not subject to the rigorous peer review that orthodox medical research papers have to undergo. This does not necessarily mean that the claims made for TM are untrue, although the British Consumers' Association has claimed that it is no better than sitting down, reading a book or just doing nothing.

The technique of TM involves sitting quietly for 20 minutes a day and reciting a secret mantra, a meaningless word designed to free your mind from the clamour of everyday thoughts. However, TM is not the only way to meditate. Meditation is simply a way of stilling the mind and there are many different ways to get there. Some involve using a mantra, others encourage the meditator to focus on an object, such as a flower, a candle or a picture, to focus on breathing (sometimes while counting), to chant, to pray, to visualize a calming scene, to reflect on a quotation or a meaningless question such as the Buddhist Koan, 'What is the sound of one hand clapping?'

People who meditate regularly usually say that they are less anxious and feel a greater sense of control over their lives. Studies show that during meditation the pulse and breathing slow, blood pressure falls and blood flow to the fingers and toes is increased. There is also a fall in the stress hormone, cortisol and the brain's electrical activity takes on a more regular rhythm known as an alpha state. It is not hard to imagine how these physiological changes might benefit someone whose arteries are narrowed or prone to go into spasm.

Although it is possible in theory to learn meditation from a book, in practice it is very difficult. If you like the idea of learning you will find a list of centres in Useful Addresses (see page 172).

RELAXATION

Interestingly, research by Harvard cardiologist Dr Herbert Benson carried out as long ago as the 1960s found that the physiological changes described above could also be brought about by a whole range of relaxation techniques including deep breathing, yoga and muscle relaxation. Such techniques are often included in rehabilitation programmes and angina management programmes. If you do not have access to such a programme they are fairly easy to learn yourself. One simple and widely used method, which involves tensing and relaxing muscles, is described below:

• Find a quiet corner where you will be undisturbed for ten minutes or so. Take the phone off the hook, loosen any tight clothing and remove your shoes.

• Now either sit comfortably or lie down with your body comfortably supported. Use cushions to support the small of your back to relieve any distracting aches and pains. Close your eyes lightly if you like.

• Starting at your feet and working your way up the rest of your body, first tense and then relax each group of muscles, paying special attention to any areas where you are usually tense.

• Clench your toes then relax them, do the same with your ankles, your thighs, your abdomen, your chest, your shoulders and your arms. Finally screw up your face and your scalp and let them relax.

• If you find during your relaxation that you are distracted by your thoughts observe them and let them go – like clouds passing over the sky.

• Concentrate on breathing slowly and evenly, breathing from your abdomen rather than your upper chest. You can check that you are breathing correctly by putting a hand on your abdomen – it should expand as you breathe in and relax as you exhale.

• After achieving a state of quiet relaxation give yourself a few moments to enjoy it then get up slowly and go about your everyday life.

Once you have become familiar with what your body feels like when it is tense you should be able to induce the relaxation response very quickly as you go about your daily life. Make it a habit to check regularly for signs of tension such as clenching your teeth, frowning, tapping your fingers or foot, hunching your shoulders and so on and then make a conscious effort to relax.

If you find it helps you may like to enrol on a de-stressing course, buy a tape or investigate a technique such as yoga or autogenic training. Relaxation should help lower blood pressure, but this should not be interpreted as lying around doing nothing all day! Physical activity (see pages 104–8) is also an important factor in the health of your heart.

CHELATION THERAPY

Another therapy which has received a lot of publicity is known as chelation. It involves infusing a chemical called EDTA (Ethylene Diamine Tetra-Acetic Acid) together with vitamins and minerals into the blood by means of a slow drip, a process that takes around three and a half hours. The EDTA bonds with heavy metals in the blood stream, allowing them to be excreted in the urine. People undergoing treament are also prescribed vitamins and minerals by mouth.

The theory behind this is that heavy metal poisoning with lead, mercury, cadmium and iron is a factor in heart disease and the development of atherosclerosis. Practitioners argue that high lead and cadmium levels are linked to high blood pressure, while an overload of iron is said to cause heart attacks. EDTA is also said to improve calcium and cholesterol metabolism by removing calcified deposits in the arteries and ridding the body of catalysts which damage cell membranes when they produce free radicals.

The UK's Arterial Heart Foundation, which offers chelation therapy, claims that 'significant levels of improvement are achieved in 88 per cent of patients'. A Danish study carried out in 1993 showed that an astonishing 89 per cent of people scheduled for heart surgery were able to avoid it after chelation. And certainly many people who have tried the therapy swear by it. Greta, who was quoted earlier, says: 'I had chronic angina and my muscle function was so poor I could hardly walk and had to be in a wheelchair. I decided to seek chelation mainly to help the myopathy (muscle weakness) which is a late complication of insulin treatment.

'After about six sessions I noticed a definite improvement in muscle function. Then I noticed I had less angina. After 20 treatments my muscle function had improved so much I was able to abandon my wheelchair. After 30 treatments I was tremendously improved. Then I decided to see how far I could go before I went downhill. In retrospect that was a mistake. I went 18 months before the symptoms took hold again, but it then took another six months of therapy. '

Chelation therapy is usually dismissed by conventional cardiologists. The Danish study was not under controlled conditions and there is still not enough evidence of chelation therapy's benefits for cardiologists to recommend it to patients. Although there are hints that it may be beginning to be taken more seriously, and the British Heart Foundation now issues a fact sheet for doctors on the therapy, Belinda Linden, nurse adviser with the Foundation says: 'It is important to keep an open mind about different treaments, but chelation therapy should not be regarded in the same light or as an alternative to established drug treatment, angioplasty or surgery.'

SUPPLEMENTARY BENEFITS

With the growing popularity of the idea among orthodox cardiologists that free radicals are involved in atherosclerosis a great deal of research is now being focused on the role of vitamin supplements in the treatment of heart disease. The ACE vitamins (not to be confused with ACE inhibitors, see Chapter 7) have received the most attention.

Certainly there is some evidence from large-scale studies carried out by well-respected researchers that vitamin E helps prevent abnormal blood clotting, increases levels of 'good' HDL cholesterol and with selenium can reduce the pain of angina. Supplementation has been found to slow the progression of atherosclerosis and the vitamin is said to reduce the tendency of arteries to close up again following angioplasty.

There is also evidence that vitamin C helps lower blood pressure and cholesterol levels, helps thin the blood and protects the lining of the arteries against further furring. Despite this, most orthodox experts still argue that not enough is known about which vitamins and minerals are most important and how they work to make any firm recommendations.

Some alternative practitioners recommend a whole range of nutritional supplements. Canadian researcher Hans R. Larsen, writing in the *International Journal of Alternative and Complementary Medicine* in August 1996, lists the following as having some research backing:

- Coenzyme Q10. An enzyme needed for the production of energy especially in the heart muscle cells. CoQ10 is said to improve the exercise capacity of people with angina, and to be useful in congestive heart failure and essential hypertension. Research is being carried out to see if CoQ10 can help people recover better from cardiac surgery.
- Magnesium. Together with calcium and potassium, magnesium is said to be effective in lowering blood pressure. On its own it is said to be useful in preventing death from heart attack and preventing further heart attacks. It is also said to reduce the frequency and severity of ventricular arrhythmias and help prevent complications after bypass surgery.
- Oils. Fish oil supplementation, according to Larsen's article, lowers blood pressure, helps prevent heart attacks and reduces the extent of restenosis in arteries opened up by angioplasty. Alpha-linolenic acid, found in flax oil and the herb purslane, helps prevent a second heart attack.
- B vitamins. Niacin (vitamin B3) is said to lower levels of 'bad' LDL cholesterol and raises levels of 'good' HDL, helps reduce atherosclerotic plaque and is said to be effective in the treatment of atrial fibrillation. It is also said to help prevent diabetes. Thiamine (vitamin B1) is said to be useful in treating congestive heart failure.
- Ginkgo. Extracts of this tree contain compounds that promote circulation. It is said to help intermittent claudication and improve the blood supply to the brain.
- Hawthorn (*Crataegus oxyacantha*) contains active compounds which dilate the blood vessels. According to Larsen it has long been used in Europe as a heart medicine. It is used to treat arrythmias, angina and high blood pressure and has been found to improve the overall function of the heart.

Other supplements that Larsen notes as having been found to help heart disease include:
- Garlic. Widely used, especially in Germany as a treatment for heart disease, research suggests that garlic supplements can lower total cholesterol and raise 'good' HDL cholesterol, lower blood pressure and have other beneficial effects on the heart and blood vessels.

- L-cartinine. This is an amino-acid-like substance that enhances the metabolism of fat in the cells, can relieve angina and improve heart function generally.

If you do decide to try out any of these supplements, ideally you should consult a qualified nutritional practitioner. As always, tell both your orthodox doctor and your complementary practitioner the full range of drugs you are taking. Supplements act on the chemistry of your blood and could react with any conventional drugs you are taking.

Bear in mind that although these supplements all have some supporting research, like most complementary treatments they have not usually undergone the stringent double-blind trial procedures applied to orthodox drugs. This is not to say that they do not work: anything which has a pharmacological action is bound to have some effect. In some cases the conventional medics are just quite rightly being cautious; in others we simply do not know enough yet one way or the other.

HEALING

Spiritual healing, through the ritual of 'laying on of hands', is as old as the human race. Barbara Rowlands, author of *The Which? Guide to Complementary Medicine* says: 'Many healers believe that the heart radiates energy and that there is far more energy coming from the heart than there is from the brain.'

Although many healers are Christians there are different sorts of healers working both within and outside the Christian church. Christians believe their healing energy is channelled through them from God, while a Chinese healer might talk about the body's own life force or *chi* and a Hindu healer might describe their healing energy as *prana*.

Some healers offer their services free and some hospitals also offer healing. If you decide to seek out a healer independently, as always you should beware of anyone who says they can cure you, especially if they are asking for a lot of money. By and large, though, healing is one the gentlest and least invasive complementary therapies and as such can be particularly useful if you are very ill. As Barbara Rowlands says, 'Healing can induce a feeling of deep relaxation which can be useful even if it only makes you feel better.'

CHAPTER 11

GETTING ON WITH YOUR LIFE

'I lead a normal life. I do voluntary work three days a week and I have an active social life.'

SYLVIA

'There are some things I don't do, but not many. I work, I play, I exercise. I enjoy food. I love, live and enjoy life.'

JOHN

HELPFUL THOUGH IT IS TO RE-EVALUATE YOUR LIFE following a diagnosis of heart disease, it is not healthy to sit around examining your navel for ever, and after a period of reflection – whether you have been in hospital or not – you will want to start getting on with the rest of your life. This chapter concentrates on the practicalities of life after heart disease, such as work, holidays and so on.

DEALING WITH WORK

Most people of working age who have heart disease are able to work. Of course, if you have been in hospital you will have needed some time off but it is encouraging to know that most people return to their previous jobs after a heart attack or surgery.

MAKING WORK LESS STRESSFUL

As part of the re-evaluation of your life it can help to think about ways in which you can make your job less stressful. We have already seen how some experts believe that there is a connection between stress at work and changes in the arteries in some people with atherosclerosis. Professor Michael Marmot, who heads the large British Whitehall Study looking at risk factors for heart disease among civil servants, has found that heart disease is especially likely to strike people who have demanding jobs over which they have little control and little support from colleagues and bosses. In a study reported in the *British Medical Journal* in 1997 he says: 'Giving employees more variety in tasks and a stronger say in decisions about work may decrease the risk of coronary heart disease.'

You might be able to speak to your boss or personnel officer to see if any changes could be made in the way you work. It can also be helpful on an individual level to look at what your job involves and think about ways of making it more enjoyable and less stressful. If you regularly find yourself saying 'Yes' when someone asks you to do something, however heavy your workload, or if you work shifts, long hours, take on a lot of overtime or regularly take work home, having a heart condition may give you the 'permission' you need to make changes for the better.

LEARNING TO PACE YOURSELF

Wherever you work it is vital to take regular breaks. If you work at a VDU you should take a break every hour to walk around and it's worth doing a few exercises to stretch your muscles.

If you have a job where you are able to control your own workload you can help yourself by learning to prioritize or put first things first. Writing down the things you have to do, planning how long they are likely to take (usually double what you imagine) and marking them in order of importance can help you keep control over your work. It can help to consider which time of day you are most alert and do jobs requiring the most concentration then, saving routine tasks for times when you feel less on the ball, such as after lunch.

Even in a job over which you have little say in your working conditions you may be able to exert control over some aspects such as the working environment. If you work in an office, for instance, you could try to make your working area more homely by placing plants and flowers on your desk, having pictures or photos of your friends and family in a place where you can see them and so on. Incidentally, keeping your desk tidy is less stressful than having unruly piles of papers that you have to rustle through every time you need to find anything.

Some people in boring or repetitive jobs such as some kinds of factory work may not be able to do much to change them, but there are ways to make work more tolerable. Talking to colleagues, listening to music while you work, taking a walk in your lunch break or simply using the time to daydream or plot what you will do during your time off are all ways of doing this.

If your job is unsatisfying, changing the way you think about it and seeing it as part of, rather than your whole life, is a useful way to reduce stress. It helps if you have to find things you enjoy doing outside work to preserve a balance between work and play. Doing something creative such as taking up painting or drawing, doing a dance class (you'll get some good aerobic exercise too), or joining an evening course provides interest and stops work being the be all and end all of life.

Clive, a civil servant, admits: 'My job doesn't interest me much but I refuse to let that get on top of me any more. I get by but the important things in my life are elsewhere. I plan my annual leave a year in advance and every three months I take some sort of break. Living in London is very stressful. I enjoy walking, so every three months I take a break in the Lake District, North Wales, Ireland, Scotland – anywhere so long as it's remote.'

RETURNING TO WORK AFTER A HEART ATTACK OR SURGERY

Just how long you need off work will depend on you, how quick your recovery is and the work that you do. Doctors usually advise waiting at least six to eight weeks after a heart attack and a similar time after surgery, but many people need longer than that. Your doctor can help you decide when you are fit to go back. By and large, if you work in an office or from home you will usually be able to return sooner than someone who has to make a long, exhausting journey or who does heavy, manual work.

Howard, who returned to his work as a lecturer three months after a heart bypass, says: 'I returned to work but because my arm was not in a sling and I did not seem obviously any different, some people did not realize what I had gone through.'

Clive returned to work six weeks after his bypass. 'I do regret going back to work so quickly. The first day back I was walking from Whitehall to Waterloo, which normally takes about 20 minutes, I got so breathless and the angina was so bad that I had to stop and hold on to the bridge.'

Such an experience, though not dangerous, can damage your confidence. Clive could have helped himself in several ways – by taking his time and pacing himself rather than trying to rush to work in the same time he had taken before his operation, by taking his angina medication before he started his walk to work or by using relaxation and breathing to help control his angina.

Some employers may agree to give you extended leave to give you time to get back to normal. Others will agree to you coming back on a part-time basis at first. If you think this would help you have a word with your boss to see if it can be arranged.

DEALING WITH COLLEAGUES

Whether you tell your colleagues about your heart condition is an individual decision only you can make. If you have had time off work your colleagues are likely to be aware you have a problem anyway. People sometimes feel reluctant to admit they have heart disease because they fear being looked upon with pity or that people will think they are not up to the demands of the job, but if you do decide to tell you will probably find people more sympathetic than you imagine. On the whole it pays to be honest because keeping things to yourself can be stressful. As Belinda Linden, nurse adviser to the British Heart Foundation says, 'It's a good idea to tell people because it puts the agenda straight. However, it can be difficult, depending on the support system within your job.'

Being open enables you to get the support you need and the camaraderie of colleagues can help you to come to terms with what has happened to you if you have had a heart attack or heart surgery. 'Sometimes I do get irritable if I've had a bad night's sleep,' says Clive. 'Some of my closer colleagues know what I've been through and they joke with me and help me laugh it off. That helps. But there are times when I feel like a freak. Even though I exercise at the heart club I can't join the fitness centre at work because if I crashed they couldn't deal with it.'

Ken, who worked as a supervisor in a store, recalls: 'People rallied round to help me. One driver would see me on the fork-lift truck and come and push me off, saying, 'Get off there. You're the one with the heart problem. We're young people – we can cope.' Taken the right way, such everyday kindnesses can be a great help in getting back to normal. On the other hand, allowing yourself to be constantly treated like an invalid or using your heart disease as an excuse to avoid doing things can be counterproductive.

CHANGING YOUR JOB

As part of the process of taking stock of your life you may decide to quit or change jobs. Some people with heart disease feel that work no longer takes such a priority and feel they want to spend more time with their families. If you don't like your job – and you can afford it – leaving or taking early retirement may be options worth considering.

John who was 36 when he had a silent heart attack and had to have bypass surgery, had worked for 18 years as a hotel chef. 'I was working split shifts, I had two broken marriages. I was completely stressed out. I'd just got remarried and I saw things with my partner slipping down the same route. I decided to get out of the hotel business. At first I did an accountancy course, but even before the results were out I realized my chances of getting a job were slim because of my age. Then my sister suggested I set up as an 'odd-job man'. I started my own business, fixing leaky washers on taps, painting, decorating, laying crazy paving, you name it I do it. I haven't looked back. It is stressful, but it's a different kind of stress because I'm the one in control.'

Mike was 56 when he had a heart bypass following a previous heart attack; he decided to take early retirement: 'I was middle management and I am convinced the pressure of that job contributed to my heart attack. I returned to work three months after surgery. Soon afterwards I was offered an attractive retirement package and decided to take it. It didn't take me long to realize, though, that I couldn't survive on my pension so I returned to work. This time I went into the voluntary sector in a consultancy position. It was a totally different atmosphere, the people I worked with were much more pleasant and the whole job far less stressful.'

Gill has also rethought her attitude to work: 'I went back to work a couple of mornings a week three months after my bypass operation. I had had complications following the bypass and I now think I tried to go back too soon. Anyway, I couldn't cope with it and as I had permanent health insurance through the company, I decided to take more time off. Now I don't think I feel like going back. My priorities have changed; I want to spend more time with my husband and doing things I like. Before, I was travelling all over place but I couldn't do that now.'

'Having a heart condition made me value life more,' Howard says. 'I took partial retirement two years ago and then last

September stopped working altogether a year early.'

If you do decide to switch jobs or give up altogether you will need to think about how to manage your finances or you might end up with extra stress. You might like to consider how you could cut down the amount you need to live on; most people can make economies if they really think about it. It is also worth thinking about alternative sources of income, such as letting out a room in your house or using other skills you have to make money.

If you are thinking about changing jobs, career counselling can be valuable in identifying your strengths and how you might apply them in other types of work. When applying for a new job it pays to be honest about your heart condition. Try to be positive and emphasize what you can do rather than what you cannot. You may be able to reassure prospective employers of your current fitness by getting a letter from your cardiologist.

HOLIDAYS AND TRAVEL

Having heart disease should not stop you going away on holiday, but it pays to plan your trip carefully so that you can enjoy your break without it being spoilt by worries about your condition.

When choosing your destination it is sensible to avoid very remote areas where it might be difficult to obtain proper medical care, high altitudes and places with extremes of temperature, whether hot or cold. Make sure you take enough tablets for the trip, as not all medications are widely available and medicines have different names in different countries so it may be hard to obtain the drug you need if you run out.

It is a good idea to inform the airline and/or the travel agent when you book that you have a heart problem. You should also make sure that you have adequate travel insurance. Go through the small print with a fine-tooth comb to find out exactly what cover is included and what exclusions there are. If you are a UK citizen form E111 from any post office entitles you to reciprocal medical care in most European countries and several others.

Reduce stress by allowing yourself plenty of time for preparation and packing, and plan your schedule carefully so that transfers can be taken leisurely. Give yourself plenty of time to recover from jet lag if you are crossing time zones. And if you are travelling around rather than staying in one resort allow yourself at least a couple of days to wind down at each new destination.

FLYING

Flying is perfectly safe for most people with coronary heart disease. Aircraft are pressurized and the air in the cabin is typically held at an altitude of around 6000ft. This pressurization allows you to breathe and move about the cabin normally no matter how high the aircraft climbs. The only time this modest pressurization may cause a problem is if you have not fully recovered from a heart attack, when it could cause breathlessness (see below).

The hustle and bustle of the airport can be stressful. Try to stay calm and avoid unwanted stress by giving yourself plenty of time to get to the airport. Once you have checked in, go through to the departure lounge where you will generally find the atmosphere is much calmer than in the rest of the airport building. Avoid carrying heavy bags by using a trolley or a bag with attached wheels. If you experience angina or breathlessness the airline may be able to arrange a porter to help you with your bags, or you can request a wheelchair or buggy.

Flying is dehydrating, which can increase the risk of thrombosis even in healthy people. To counteract dehydration make sure you drink plenty of fluids – plain, non-sparkling mineral water is the best choice, as alcohol is dehydrating and carbonated drinks increase the gas expansion caused by ascent.

During flights of over two hours you should try to take a turn up and down the cabin from time to time, as sitting in the same position for any length of time encourages swelling of the feet and legs and stagnation of blood flow in the legs, which can cause deep vein thrombosis. If you cannot walk in the aisle circle your ankles and raise your toes with the heels on the ground every half hour to prevent sluggish circulation.

AFTER A HEART ATTACK OR SURGERY

Provided your condition is stable and you no longer need constant medical supervision there is no reason why you shouldn't go away on holiday. Most airlines allow you to travel ten days after a heart attack provided you can briskly walk 100 yards on the flat without chest pain or undue breathlessness. However, the British Heart Foundation advises, 'Travel is best delayed for about six weeks after a heart attack or longer in patients who have heart failure or severe angina.' Your doctor will be able to help you decide whether travelling is advisable.

You should contact the airline medical department well before you are due to go if you would like their medical team to provide a wheelchair or assistance with early boarding, and ensure that you get any care you need during the flight. You should also get a medical questionnaire from the airline office when you book your ticket, which your family doctor should fill in and return to the airline so any special provisions can be made for your journey.

Once at your destination, try to pace yourself. There is no need to spend every minute sitting under a beach umbrella but it is not a good idea to plan vigorous activities every second of the day either. Belinda Linden, nurse adviser with the British Heart Foundation advises, 'It is a good idea to build up your stamina before you go so that you can do what you want to do while you are on holiday.'

Above all try to maintain an optimistic attitude. Howard, who has had a heart bypass, says: 'I don't like to sit around on holiday and after my bypass I continued to take active holidays. I was able to send a card to my consultant saying I'd climbed 100-odd steps.' Clive takes regular walking holidays both in the UK and abroad. 'I can appreciate that people who have lost confidence after surgery could worry,' he says, 'but going away in that frame of mind is no use. The main thing for me is not to take chances. I get guidebooks before I go and plan my walks. I tend to steer clear of the more strenuous ones and go for those marked easy/moderate. I make sure I have proper boots and equipment and wet-weather gear, and that I tell people where I'm going.'

If you are going somewhere sunny and have had heart surgery you should use a total sun block on your scar as the sun dampens down the activity of the immune system in the skin and this can impede healing.

For further advice about health on holiday, *Stay Healthy Abroad* by Rob Ryan is published by the Health Education Authority.

DRIVING

Ordinary driving should present no problem if you have a heart condition. However, if you develop angina while driving or suffer with unstable angina you should tell the doctor and inform the Driving Vehicle Licence Agencies (DVLA), as you may have to stop driving until your condition is under control. In the UK ask for leaflet DVLA D100 at the post office.

AFTER A HEART ATTACK OR SURGERY

In the UK the DVLA recommends that you should not drive for four weeks after a heart attack; most surgeons advise waiting around six weeks. Immediately after a heart operation your chest is likely to be sore. Driving can put pressure on your shoulders and chest wound and wearing a seat belt can also be uncomfortable. You do not need to inform the DVLA if you have had a heart attack or heart operation unless you have been left with any complications such as angina that occur while driving. You should, however, inform your insurance company in case there are any restrictions on your policy.

Once any statutory requirements have been met it is very much up to you when you feel fit to get back behind the wheel. Your doctor can advise you and you should also be guided by how well you feel. It can take a little while to regain confidence behind the wheel – take it easy at first and don't expect too much of yourself. It makes sense to limit your trips to short runs when you first get back into the driving seat and to avoid busy times of day and heavy traffic. It can sometimes be a good idea to ask your partner or a friend to accompany you on your first few trips out until you regain your confidence on the road. If you are on medication or your condition is not straightforward, have a word with your doctor before resuming driving.

IF DRIVING IS YOUR JOB

In the UK there are special rules applying to re-licensing of drivers with professional or vocational driving licences (PCV or LGV). You can get a copy of these from the DVLA. You may be permitted to drive after three months provided you have completed a standard treadmill test without experiencing any heart symptoms.

MONEY, MONEY, MONEY

Heart disease can have an impact on your financial situation that extends far beyond any time you may have to have off work.

'Money concerns are often a major concern for men who are the main breadwinners, partly because they may feel that their job is on the line, or for self-employed people. This is a pity because it adds to anxieties about the future,' says Belinda Linden.

As with any worry, facing up to your situation can help you to feel easier. If you anticipate having problems with regular payments such as your mortgage, it is a good idea to make appointments with your bank and building society managers to try and work out a solution before you start missing payments. It is usually also possible to make arrangements to pay bills by smaller instalments over a period of time.

However worrying you find the prospect of facing up to monetary difficulties, the very worst thing you can do is bury your head in the sand. If you need help or advice about money, Citizens Advice Bureaux have specially trained advisers who can help you sort out your finances and sometimes even write on your behalf to any people to whom you owe money.

INSURANCE MATTERS

Insurance can sometimes be an issue for people who have heart disease. If you already had a life assurance policy when you were diagnosed with heart disease you should be covered, so long as you did not conceal information on the original application form. If you are taking out a new policy or changing your policy you may sometimes experience some difficulties. There may also be changes to your motoring insurance policy and this too may be an area of difficulty.

'Although some companies are receptive and supportive, some are unhelpful and premiums are sometimes enormously high, especially if someone has undergone surgery,' observes Belinda Linden. 'This can be very unfair, especially when patients have often made efforts to change their lifestyle and feel as a result that their health has improved so much.'

Be that as it may it can be helpful to prepare yourself for some rejections and try not to take them personally. The British Heart Foundation has a list of sympathetic insurance companies.

CLAIMING BENEFITS

Although most people with heart disease continue to work, a few may find that they are prevented either temporarily or permanently. If you have to have time off work or cannot work because of your heart disease you may be entitled to certain benefits. In the UK you can claim Statutory Sick Pay for up to 28 weeks after being laid off sick. After this you may be eligible for Short-term Incapacity Benefit for up to 28 weeks. After this Incapacity Benefit can be paid at the long-term, slightly higher rate. You should be able to top up a low income with Income Support. How much you get will depend on your exact situation at the time that you make your claim and whether you or your partner have any income or savings.

If your condition is such that you need personal care or have problems with mobility you may be entitled to Disability Living Allowance. You may also be entitled to certain rights and considerations under the UK's Disability Discrimination Act which came in between 1995 and 1997. According to the Act disability is any 'physical or mental impairment which has a substantial and long-term adverse effect on a person's ability to carry out normal day-to-day activities'. Long-term effects are considered to be those that have lasted at least 12 months, or are likely to last at least 12 months. As an example of how the Act may affect you, your employer is not allowed to dismiss you because you are sometimes off work as a result of your heart disease if the time you take off is little more than what the employer accepts as sick leave for other employees. However, this does not apply if you work for a company with fewer than 20 employees.

The benefits system is complicated and it can be difficult to find your way around. 'Many people don't draw the benefits they are entitled to because they are not aware they are entitled to them,' says Belinda Linden. 'People sometimes have to go through hoops to get benefits because the goal posts are constantly being changed. The key thing is to keep persevering and not to give up. It also helps to keep a photocopy of any forms you have filled in and letters you have sent.'

The rules for drawing benefits change quite frequently too, so it is worth making sure you have up-to-date advice by contacting your local Department of Social Security or Citizens Advice Bureau. You can get written guidelines on applying for benefits from the Department of Health (see Useful Addresses). There is also a Benefits Enquiry Line, which can give general advice on your eligibility for benefits. The Disability Alliance also gives information on benefits and publishes a handbook which contains useful information. In the US the American Heart Foundation should be able to help you.

CHAPTER 12

MOVING ON

CAROLYN, TWO YEARS AFTER DEVELOPING ANGINA
AND HAVING STENTS INSERTED:

'I was always one for visiting everyone. Now I tend to do half the visiting I used to and let them come to me. I've never been completely laid back because I like to be everybody's friend. Having heart disease has forced me to slow my pace down and think of myself and what I want more. I do still think about it and it has taken me a lot of time to regain my confidence. I'm not religious but sometimes I wake up in the morning and I thank God I'm still here.'

CLIVE, FOUR YEARS AFTER A HEART ATTACK:

'It has forced me to change. I think I'm a better person now. Being part of the support group made me realize that there is always someone who is in a worse situation than you are. Feeling the support of other people who have been through the same thing is very important to me.'

GILL, TWO YEARS AFTER BEING DIAGNOSED WITH
A BLOCKED AORTA AND HAVING A BYPASS:

'If you had talked to me six months ago I would have been much less positive. Today I feel much better. It's made me a much wiser person. It's also put a completely different aspect on life. I'm more selfish, I suppose because I might not be here tomorrow. It's made me realize you only live once – this isn't a rehearsal. We travel more now. I think if I hadn't had heart disease we would have saved our money for the grandchildren.'

GRETA, WHO HAS WIDESPREAD ARTERIAL DISEASE DUE TO DIABETES,
11 YEARS AFTER A BYPASS:

'It's never likely to go away altogether but life is much more tolerable. I am able to live a more reasonable lifestyle.'

HOWARD, FIVE YEARS AFTER DEVELOPING ANGINA
AND TWO YEARS AFTER A QUADRUPLE BYPASS:

'You've got to have an intelligent approach to it. I value life more today. I am very highly strung but I've made a conscious effort not to let things upset me so much. I surprise myself now by all the things I used to do and the committees I attended.'

JIM, TEN YEARS AFTER A HEART ATTACK AND EIGHT YEARS
AFTER A TRIPLE BYPASS:

'I believe it is important to think positive. I never looked back. Some people I've met won't believe they can get better. I do voluntary work at the hospital, I run and I enjoy life. There are still lots of things I want and intend to do.'

JOHN, 11 YEARS AFTER DIAGNOSIS AND FOLLOWING
TWO HEART BYPASSES:

'I recognize my limitations. I'll go up and down a ladder but I'll draw a line at certain things. I love, live and enjoy life. I don't feel as if I'm on borrowed time, I feel as if I've been given a whole new lease of life.'

KEN, 15 YEARS AFTER A HEART ATTACK
AND SEVEN AFTER A BYPASS:

'I did get depressed at first but I'm ex-Navy and I think it's important to think positive: you can't have low moral fibre. I took voluntary redundancy last year and my wife and I both go to the cardiac exercise group. We both get something out of it, it's an evening out of the house and we're both much fitter.'

LEN, 34 YEARS AFTER A HEART ATTACK, 13 YEARS AFTER A BYPASS AND
10 YEARS AFTER HAVING A PACEMAKER:

'I feel I was reborn when I had my bypass. It gives you a second chance to re-evaluate your life, to live a cleaner life, to take hold of life and not let life take hold of you.'

MIKE, SEVEN YEARS AFTER THE FIRST OF TWO HEART ATTACKS AND
A BYPASS:

'No one thinks about having a heart attack until they have one. It's such a jolt, not just to you but to your partner. After the second attack I felt as if the bottom had fallen out of my world. You can no longer control your own life. You can't earn any money. A lot of people turn their back on you. It's a real kick in the pants. Now I try to take each day as it comes. If your body's saying rest, you have to rest. I get bad days when my breathing is bad, and I've got pain in my chest and tingling. Other days I feel terrific. It's a question of learning to take life more as it comes. Most heart patients are very active – I still find it hard to slow down but I read a lot, watch TV, listen to music.'

PETER, 12 YEARS AFTER BEING DIAGNOSED WITH ANGINA AND SEVEN
AFTER HAVING A BYPASS:

'I'd never been a smoker and I'd never had a bad diet, my wife and I were never into fried foods. So I was bitterly disappointed when I developed heart disease, but I'm convinced I made a far better recovery because of my healthy lifestyle. I also think it makes a difference to be confident. You've got to trust and rely on the surgeons.'

SYLVIA, NINE YEARS AFTER BEING DIAGNOSED WITH ANGINA AND THREE
AFTER A BYPASS:

'I'm very lucky because I'm positive-minded and that has got me through. When I'm walking up hill it kills me and wind is the worst thing in the world, but otherwise I lead a normal life. I don't sit back and let it get the better of me. The doctor at the hospital made me feel as though I can carry on, and you can. I'm 77 today and I still feel good. I feel very grateful.'

Appendix 1

What To Do in an Emergency

The following action plan is based on advice contained in the British Heart Foundation's booklet *Living with Heart Disease*:

STEP ONE
Is it a heart attack or angina?
If the pain is bearable, then rest. If you have been prescribed pills or spray for angina, use them now. If the pain goes away after 15 minutes rest and/or after taking the pills, it may have been angina. If the pain is unusually severe phone your doctor and tell him your symptoms.

Is it a heart attack or indigestion?
If you do suffer from indigestion and have an attack that lasts for more than 15 minutes despite taking your usual tablets, then phone your doctor.

STEP TWO
Getting help
Phone your doctor and tell him your symptoms.

Dial 999
- if the doctor can't be contacted after five minutes
- if the doctor is coming but the pain suddenly becomes much worse
- if the doctor is coming but you feel you are about to pass out – ask for an ambulance. Tell them it is a suspected heart attack, then go to Step Three.

If you can't get to a telephone get someone to drive you to the nearest hospital. DON'T DRIVE YOURSELF.

STEP THREE
Waiting for help
Make sure the door at home is left unlocked. Sit back in a comfortable position and wait for the doctor or ambulance.

CPR (CARDIOPULMONARY RESUSCITATION)

Reading how to do CPR in a book is better than nothing, but you will feel much more confident and be able to administer it more effectively if you learn how to do it properly. If a member of your family has a heart condition it is well worth taking a course in CPR so that you can be prepared in case of an emergency. Every responsible member of your family should learn to recognize the warning signs and know what to do in an emergency. The British Heart Foundation recommends the following action:

Assessment	Approach the person with care. Try to ascertain if the person is conscious by gentle shaking and shouting 'Are you OK?' If he or she does not respond, call for help.
Airway	Open the airway by tilting the head back and lifting the chin.
Breathing	Look, listen and feel for signs of breathing.
Circulation	Feel for the pulse in the neck just to the side of the windpipe.

If the person is unconscious, has stopped breathing and has no pulse:

- Call for an ambulance, then position the person on their back on the floor. Open airway again.
- Use the same method as before. Give two of your own breaths to the person. Close their nostrils with your finger/thumb and blow into the mouth, making sure that the mouth is sealed so no air escapes. The person's chest should expand.
- Perform 15 chest compressions. Find the notch at the bottom of the breastbone. Measure two finger widths above this. Place both hands on the breastbone. Press down firmly and smoothly 15 times at about 80 times a minute.
- Repeat two breaths, then 15 compressions. Continue until professional help arrives.
- If the person is unconscious and not breathing but a pulse is present, give ten breaths. If the person still does not respond call an ambulance, then re-assess.

APPENDIX 2
PRESCRIBED DRUGS AND THEIR SIDE EFFECTS

HEART DRUGS AT A GLANCE

Condition	Drugs often prescribed
Angina	Nitrates; beta-blockers; calcium-channel blockers; aspirin
Heart attack	Thrombolytics (clotbusters); aspirin; beta-blockers. Other drugs may be prescribed in more complicated cases
High blood pressure	Diuretics; beta-blockers; calcium-channel blockers; ACE inhibitors are the main ones. Others include clonidine; hydralazine; methyldopa; minoxidil; alpha-blockers
Heart failure	Diuretics; ACE inhibitors; digoxin
Disorders of heart rhythm	Anti-arrhythmic drugs
Secondary prevention (i.e drugs used to correct risk factors for heart disease)	Cholesterol-lowering drugs; blood-pressure-lowering drugs; aspirin

WHICH LIPID-LOWERING DRUG?

Drug group	How taken	Possible side effects
Resins (cholestyramine; colestipol)	As granules mixed with water or fruit juice	Stomach discomfort, heartburn, constipation
Fibrates (clofibrate; gemfibrozil; fenofibrate; bezafibrate)	With meals	Nausea, stomach upsets, muscle pains
Nicotinic acid (nicofuranose; acipimox)		Flushing and faintness on first use; headache (which can be counteracted by aspirin); itching
Statins (simvastatin; pravastatin)		Stomach upsets; muscle pains; weakness. Statins can interact with fibrates to cause severe muscle pain

Useful Addresses

Heart organizations
UK
British Heart Foundation
14 Fitzhardinge Street
London WlH 4DH
0171 935 0185
Information line: 0990 200656

National Heart Forum
Tavistock House South
Tavistock Square
London WC1H 9LG
0171 383 7638

British Cardiac Patients
    Association (Zipper Club)
6 Rampton End
Willingham
Cambs CB4 5JB
01954 202022

Family Heart Association
    (patient information charity
    specializing in blood lipid
    disorders, including inherited
    high cholesterol)
7 North Road
Maidenhead
Berks SL6 1PL
01628 28638

USA
American Heart Association
National Center
7272 Greenville Avenue
Dallas TX 75231-4596
Information line: 1-800 AHA
USA1 (1-800 242 8721)

Australia
National Heart Foundation of
    Australia
Corner of Denman Street
Geils Court
Deakin
ACT 2600
616 282 2144

Canada
Heart and Stroke Foundation
    of Canada
160 George Street
Suite 200
Ottawa
Ontario K1N 9MZ
1613 241 4361

New Zealand
National Heart Foundation of
    New Zealand
17 Great South Road
Newmarket
PO Box 17–160
Greenlane
Auckland 5
6495 24 6005

Quit-Smoking Organizations
ASH (Action on Smoking
    and Health)
109 Gloucester Place
London WlH 3PH
0171 935 3519

QUIT
Victory House
Tottenham Court Road
London WlP 0HA
0171 388 5775

Complementary Therapies
Institute for Complementary
  Medicine
PO Box 194
London SE16 1QZ
0171 237 5165

Transcendental Meditation
Beacon House
Willow Walk
Skelmersdale
Lancs WN8 6UR
0990 143733

Arterial Disease Clinic
  (chelation therapy)
3rd Floor, 571 Wimpole Street
London W1M 7DF
0171 486 1095
  and
70 The Avenue
Leigh
Lancs WN7 1ET
01942 676617

Department of Health
PO Box 410
Wetherby
Yorks LS23 7LN
Benefits enquiry line:
0800 882200

FURTHER READING

These are all books that you might find helpful to read. Some are technical, others will give you ideas on how to change your lifestyle. One or two are out of print so you might have to order them from a library.

The Coronary Prevention Group, *Preventing Heart Disease*, The
  Consumers' Association and Hodder & Stoughton, 1991
Julian, Dr Desmond and Marley, Claire, *Coronary Heart Disease:
  The Facts*, Oxford University Press, 1991
Litvinoff, Sarah, *The Relate Guide to Better Relationships*, Ebury Press,
  1991
Marieb, Elaine N., *Human Anatomy and Physiology*, Benjamin
  Cummings Publishing Company Inc., 1995
Pietroni, Patrick, *Holistic Living*, J. M. Dent and Sons, 1986
Rowlands, Barbara, *The* Which? *Guide to Complementary Medicine*,
  Consumers' Association, 1996
Vaughan, Sue, *Finding the Stillness Within a Busy World*, C. W. Daniel
  Company, 1995
Zaret, Barry L; Moser, Marvin; Cohen, Lawrence S. (editors), *Yale
  University School of Medicine Heart Book*, Hearst Books, 1992

INDEX